Pediatric Ethics

Monographs in Clinical Pediatrics

This series is one for all professionals concerned with child health and disease. It covers a number of clinically relevant topics, with each monograph dealing with a specific theme or disease entity. Volumes are oriented toward practical aspects of clinical pediatrics, but contain sufficient basic science to enable the reader to understand the logical basis for the subject under discussion. Common clinical problems are covered and controversies are highlighted, providing authoritative guidance for the investigation and management of diseases seen in pediatric practice.

Volume 1: *Essential Pediatric Dermatology*
by James A. Keipert

Volume 2: *Infectious Diseases in Pregnancy and the Newborn Infant*
by Gwendolyn L. Gilbert

Volume 3: *Pediatric Neuro-Oncology: New Trends in Clinical Research*
edited by Roger J. Packer, W. Archie Bleyer and Carl Pochedly

Volume 4: *Atherosclerosis Prevention: Identification and Treatment of the Child with High Cholesterol*
edited by Marc S. Jacobson

Volume 5: *Feeding Problems and Eating Disorders in Children and Adolescents*
edited by Peter J. Cooper and Alan Stein

Volume 6: *Depression in Children and Adolescents*
edited by Harold S. Koplewicz and Emily Klass

Volume 7: *Adolescent Medicine*
edited by I. Ronald Shenker

Volume 8: *Inflammatory Bowel Disease in Children and Adolescents*
edited by Jeremiah J. Levine and Michael J. Pettei

Volume 9: *Pediatric Ethics — from Principles to Practice*
edited by Robert C. Cassidy and Alan R. Fleischman

This book is part of a series. The publisher will accept continuation orders which may be cancelled at any time and which provide for automatic billing and shipping of each title in the series upon publication. Please write for details.

Pediatric Ethics
From Principles to Practice

Edited by

Robert C. Cassidy

Schneider Children's Hospital
Long Island Jewish Medical Center
New York, USA

and

Alan R. Fleischman

The New York Academy of Medicine
New York, USA

harwood academic publishers
Australia • Canada • China • France • Germany • India • Japan • Luxembourg
Malaysia • The Netherlands • Russia • Singapore • Switzerland • Thailand
United Kingdom

Emmaplein 5
1075 AW Amsterdam
The Netherlands

British Library Cataloguing in Publication Data

Pediatric ethics : from principles to practice.
(Monographs in clinical pediatrics ; v. 9)
1. Pediatrics – Moral and ethical aspects 2. Medical ethics
I. Cassidy, Robert C. II. Fleischman, Alan R.
174.2

ISBN 3718657562

Contents

Preface

This is a book for pediatric practitioners, written by experienced pediatric caregivers. It targets the most serious and prevalent ethical issues that pediatric caregivers confront. It has been specifically designed to enhance the practitioner's ability to identify, evaluate and decide how to manage the real ethical challenges that arise in caring for children and their families. *Pediatric Ethics: from Principles to Practice* is dedicated to empowering the practicing clinician to make more thoughtful judgements when faced with difficult ethical dilemmas.

As the title emphasizes, we have attempted to demonstrate how individual judgements should be developed by a systematic process of disciplined deliberation grounded on fundamental values. For each issue, practical examples, close order analysis, and step-by-step explanations of judgements are provided. Our first chapter, "From Principles to Practice", is specifically designed to demonstrate and explain the systemic standards of such disciplined ethical judgement.

Chapters 2 and 3 both deal with the agonizing issues arising in life-or-death decisions. Chapter 2 reviews the history of ethical, legal and professional reflection on this critical issue. Chapter 3 demonstrates how a practicing neonatologist melds these traditions with his own individual sensitivity and experience. Together they demonstrate how the individual practitioner's judgement is strengthened by reasoning in dialogue with the community of concerned colleagues.

The remaining chapters apply the principles of disciplined judgement and the spirit of collegial dialogue to the full range of ethical issues across the broad spectrum of pediatric care. From the tragic questions of critical care to the most common ethical undercurrents in primary care – from truth-telling for the child to confidentiality for the adolescent – from the problem of 'using' children for research to the issue of 'using' families for home care – from 'futility' in intensive care to conflicting interests in the private office – all the most difficult and challenging pediatric issues are faced.

In sum, our primary purpose has been to provide a dialogue with experienced, sensitive and reflective colleagues engaged in the practice of ethical decision-making – and to demonstrate for practitioners how to use that discipline in caring for children and families.

List of Contributors

Jeffrey Blustein
Mercy College
Albert Einstein College of Medicine
Jack D. Weiler Hospital
1825 Eastchester Rd.
Bronx, New York 10461

Jeffrey Burns
Boston Children's Hospital
300 Longwood Avenue
Boston
Massachusetts 02115
U.S.A.

Robert C. Cassidy
Schneider Children's Hospital
Long Island Jewish Medical Center
New Hyde Park
New York 11040
U.S.A.

Alan R. Fleischman
Senior Vice President
The New York Academy of Medicine
1216 Fifth Avenue
New York 10029
U.S.A.

Joel E. Frader
Children's Hospital of Pittsburgh
3705 Fifth Avenue at DeSoto Street
Pittsburgh
Pennsylvania 15213
U.S.A.

Susan Grobman
The Children's Health Fund
317 East 64th Street
New York 10021
U.S.A.

Sanford Leikin
Children's Hospital
National Medical Center
111 Michigan Avenue N
Washington D.C. 20010
U.S.A.

Ruth Macklin
Albert Einstein College of Medicine
1300 Morris Park Avenue
Bronx
New York 10461
U.S.A.

Andrew P. Mezey
Albert Einstein College of Medicine
1300 Morris Park Avenue
Bronx
New York 10461
U.S.A.

Jonathan D. Moreno
SUNY Health Science Center at Brooklyn
450 Clarkson Avenue, Box 116
Brooklyn
New York 11203
U.S.A.

Alex Okun
Albert Einstein College of Medicine
1300 Morris Park Avenue
Bronx
New York 10461
U.S.A.

Irwin Redlener
The Children's Health Fund
317 East 64th Street
New York 10021
U.S.A.

Cindy H. Rushton
Johns Hopkins Children's Center
600 N. Wolfe St.
Baltimore
Maryland 21205
U.S.A.

Robert Truog
Boston Children's Hospital
300 Longwood Avenue
Boston
Massachusetts 02115
U.S.A.

Gary A. Walco
Tomorrow's Children's Institute
Hackensack Medical Center
30 Prospect Avenue
Hackensack
New Jersey 07601
U.S.A.

1 From Principles to Practice

Robert C. Cassidy

Schneider Children's Hospital, Long Island Jewish Medical Center, 269–01 76th Avenue, New Hyde Park, New York 11040, USA

INTRODUCTION: ETHICS — A MATTER OF JUDGEMENT

> The mother of a 13-year-old boy is worried that he may be using drugs. She believes it appropriate for the pediatrician to test him without his knowledge or consent. The pediatrician believes that such a violation of the boy's privacy is not ethically justified — Who's right?
>
> A premature infant has suffered severe neurological damage from an intraventricular hemorrhage. The parents demand an end to life support. The nurse coordinator insists we must continue, and the pediatrician is ambivalent — Who's right?
>
> A 12-year-old leukemic has not responded to treatment and is terminal. The pediatrician believes the young person should be told. But, the parents are adamantly opposed — Who's right?
>
> After 2 years with a pediatrician, a mother of three children has just lost her job-related insurance and gone on Medicaid. The doctor decides to discharge her as his patient. His receptionist is outraged — Who's right?

These are ethical issues. They are just a few examples of the ethical problems that all too frequently confront caregivers in pediatric practice. One way or another, they must be decided. But which way is right? Who is to say?

The purpose of this whole volume, and especially of this chapter, is to help practitioners deal with these questions *better*. Note the emphasis: this is not an answer book, offering *right* answers. *Rather*, it is designed to help practitioners produce *better* answers to the ethical questions they face in their offices, clinics, and hospitals.

But, are some answers better than others? Yes, we believe so. As we shall argue in the next section, ethics is a matter of judgement. It is true that the answers to ethical questions do not have the self-evident objectivity of matters-of-fact. But, neither do they permit the self-indulgent anarchy of mere matters-of-opinion. As Dr. Howard Brody has stated:

> Ethics is the study of the rational process for determining the best course of action in the face of conflicting choices.[1]

As a rational process, ethics is a matter of judgement. It is a matter of judgement whether truth-telling or confidentiality or foregoing life-extending treatment is appropriate in a particular case. And, as with clinical judgement and judicial judgement, judgements are better if the judges are better — more knowledgeable, more critical, and more disciplined, for example.

In order to articulate the standards for that rational process of judgement, we shall first ask the question, "If we were writing a job description for a good judge, what would be the essential qualifications?" Next, we shall analyze the nature of the *ethical problems* that require our best judgement. Then, we shall outline how *ethical answers* have traditionally been developed, concentrating on the *grounds* invoked to give authority to individual reasonings. Finally, we shall provide a set of procedural *tests*, to help us be assured that we have produced our best possible judgements.

GOOD JUDGES

Judgement is the required task for practical ethics. Therefore, we can employ the qualities of a "good judge" to design the model for the practice of ethics. The important point is that this is a discriminating standard. It can be used to distinguish between the ethical judgements of various persons, just as we would between the judgements of judges in a court, or at a musical competition, or for an athletic match.

In all these situations there are standards of good (and bad) judging. These same standards should be applied to all who would claim the high office of judges of the ethical issues in medical care.

Before laying out these performative standards, consider just two practical examples. If a judgement were to be made about whether to tell an 11-year-old leukemic that she was dying, persons who allowed their own interests to compromise their judgements of the child's best interests should be regarded as less qualified to judge. Or, if we were judging whether we should continue life-support on a newborn after a grade IV intraventricular hemorrhage, persons who knew the prognostic data should be regarded as better qualified to judge. The parents of one damaged newborn expressed just such concerns:

> We wonder whether parents of defective newborns are ever in a position to determine what is best for their child because of their emotional state, lack of knowledge and information and inherent conflicts of interest.[2]

They also, we should note, raised similar concerns about the doctors' judgements, given their apparent inconsistency and potential self-interests. (For a more specific discussion of this point, see Chapter 3.)

What, then, are the qualities that justify recognizing the authority of someone to make bioethical judgements?

1. Knowledgeable

Good bioethical judges are knowledgeable in three important ways. First, they must be aware of, and understand, the pertinent medical facts, including the full diagnostic and prognostic picture and the relevant elements of all significant options. The information necessary for a valid informed consent sets an appropriate standard. Informed judges must fully comprehend the given situation. And, they must know the nature of each choice: its purpose, its risks and benefits, and the probability of both. All this must be based on the disciplined command of the best available sources of the most accurate and complete information.

Second, good judges must be educated in the substantive standards of their profession. Judging should be a communal activity, in which an individual applies the accumulated experience and wisdom of a professional community to a specific situation. The precedents, procedural rules, protocols and other criteria crafted within a tradition must be known, and used, either as received, or as modified with craftsmanlike care.

Third, knowledgeable judges must be serious students of the responsible critics of their community and its traditions, and of their own personal dispositions, interests and judgements. Defensive insularity is a fault. An openness to well-honed challenges from others and a willingness to be self-challenging are virtues.

As an example, assume you have a 16-year-old hemophiliac who is HIV^{+} and has a sexual partner. What do you need to know before deciding whether to warn the third party? First, information, for example the routes and probabilities of transmission of HIV; Second, the tradition of professional confidentiality from Hippocrates down through contemporary codes of ethics of professional guilds; Third, the critical challenges to professional confidentiality developed in recent court decisions. Competent judges must command all the pertinent material in these categories.

2. Impartial

Good judges are impartial in two senses of the term. First, they are disinterested. That is, they do not stand to gain from any particular choice. Especially in pediatrics, where the judges are so often making a surrogate decision about the best interests of a child, it is essential that the interests of the judges do not create a conflict with those of the child.

Second, they are open-minded, which means that they have not pre-judged the case and foreclosed options before a full and balanced evaluation. Parents overwhelmed by the burdens of caring for a handicapped child exemplify a serious potential for a disqualifying conflict-of-interest. A neo-natologist reflexively committed to unqualified heroic efforts for every newborn is an example of a similarly close-minded attitude.

3. Systematic

This requirement is also two-fold: First, to be orderly. The process by which the good judge decides is consistent, coherent and comprehensive. Decisions can be clearly seen to be the products of a definable, defensible, and sequential process of analysis, deliberation and closure. Second, to be disciplined. She or he knows and accepts the rules of the system. R. M. Hare of Oxford titled a book *Freedom or Reason*, by which he meant that those who accept the rules of rational thought are no longer free to choose as they might wish. Good judges do not allow themselves the freedom of ungrounded and undisciplined answers, no matter how satisfying. Good judges are good servants of the laws of judgement, including the requirements of accurate analysis and rational deliberation.

We have mentioned "consistent" as an element of thinking, i.e., using terms with the same meaning and force in similar circumstances. There is, however, a more fundamental sense of consistency, which becomes a matter of fairness. It is seen in the judge who reaches similar conclusions given similar cases. This, of course, does not call for an overly rigid uniformity of judgement. But, it does mean that equals should receive equal treatment, and that exceptions to rules should be based on defined and justified rules for such exceptions.

As an example, assume we have two new admissions in the Emergency Room waiting to be worked up. The basic rule might be "First come, first served". But the rule of exceptions would authorize us to take the more critically ill first, justifying the exception as sacrificing a lesser good for the sake of a greater good. But, what if one child is "well-connected"? It is questionable whether the good judge would allow an economic exception to the therapeutically grounded rules of clinical triage. Any such exception would have to meet a very heavy burden of proof to be ethically justifiable.

4. Decisive

The task is to work systematically through the complicated elements of a complex question and to come out with an answer, a judgement, at the end of that process. The competent judge is able to achieve closure. The qualified judge is able to meet the challenge of "The buck stops here".

5. Corrigible

On the other hand, the process of judgement must constantly be used against its own products. New information, new arguments, or new experiences may, indeed must, be utilized to challenge previous positions in an on-going process of reflection and reform.

6. Empathetic

Empathy is a way of knowing other persons, a way of appreciating their personal sense of self and of the significance of self, even when their nature or needs or views are radically different from one's own. Breadth of sensitivity creates a breadth of understanding of others. This in turn grounds a depth of concern and respect for others and their diverse, often opposing, positions. This final qualification signals the good judge as a responsive and responsible member of the complex community of human individuals with their diverse interests, values and commitments. It marks those who, while formulating their individual judgements with disciplined integrity, are also committed to making our ethical world safe for diversity.

Our next concern is to analyze the nature of the problems that ethical judges are responsible for. We shall then be in a position to tackle the final, and most difficult question, "What is the appropriate process for producing the best possible answers?", also known as the most judicious judgements.

WHAT IS AN ETHICAL PROBLEM? A DILEMMA

> I wish someone would bring me a one-armed expert, so the s.o.b. couldn't say, 'But, on the other hand .....'
>
> paraphrase of Harry S. Truman

Practical ethics is about problem-solving. Very simply, we could say it is the process by which we attempt to find the best answer to the following sort of problem: In this situation (A), for this person (B), what is the best/right thing to do (C)? For example: A specialist has injured a child you referred to him and refuses to tell the parents the truth. As the family's pediatrician, what should you do?

Notice a couple of obvious but important elements of this model problem. First, it begins with a very specific situation. Our focus in what we could call "practitioner ethics" is very limited, very specific, very individual. This, as we are all aware, means that our answers will have to be limited, specific and individual. As George Eliot put it in *The Mill on the Floss*, "Moral judgements must remain false and hollow unless they are checked and enlightened by perpetual reference to the special circumstances that mark the individual lot."[3]

Checking on our example, our problem (and, hence, our answer) would be quite different if you were, say, a resident, and not the family's physician. Our problem/answer might also be affected by other factors, such as how serious the injury is. We shall highlight these "tilt factors" later in this chapter. For now, we just need to register the "circumstantial" nature of practical ethical problems.

But, does that mean that our problems and consequent answers are purely circumstantial? And, that, since the circumstances are always individual, that our answers can only be equally individual, such that no general values or ordering rules could be applicable?

Yes — and No! Yes, our answers must be aware of and responsive to the individuality of the real situations. But, that does not mean they end up completely idiosyncratic, with no order to our understanding and no standards to our judging. A parallel? The practice of medical judgement. Obviously each patient is different. But, "different" makes sense to the physician as different from an identifiable standard. A particular 6-year-old boy is the height he is. He is "different". But, his individual height is locatable on a general scale of physical development. And, if the physician were to decide to treat the child with growth hormone, the correct dosage would be titrated to fit the individual child. But, the titration would be according to definable and defensible rules of calculated adjustment.

I put it to you, as our British colleagues would say, that the practice of ethics, like the practice of medicine, consists of knowing two things: (1) the basic nature of the problem and the relevant individuating factors, and (2) the basic nature of the solutions and the relevant rules for applying them properly to the properly individuated problem.

Now, go back to our model of ethical problem-solving. There is one other element besides its orderly specificity that we must highlight. It is that these problems are "ethical". What does that mean? To completely answer the question, "What is ethical?" would require an enormous investment of time and effort. We would have to study the last 2500 years of secular and religious moral philosophy about the nature of good and evil, right and wrong, and the standards of moral behavior from Aristotle and Plato down through Mill and Kant to Ramsey and Rawls.

But, for our purpose, which is to give structure to the practitioner's practice of ethics, the question we need to answer is more limited, more targeted. It is "What is the nature of an ethical problem?" Once we have identified the logic of the problems we have to deal with, we will be able to choose the right logical instruments to deal with them.

So, what is the nature of an ethical problem? In a word, it is a "*dilemma*". Recall our problematic example: Should you tell the parents about your colleague's error? Put yourself in that situation and feel the rhythm. Note how you are pulled in two opposing directions. On the one hand may be your sense of an obligation to be honest with your patients/parents and your concern that your patient receive appropriate compensation, amongst other factors. But, on the other hand, there may be your loyalty to a colleague, and your concern about the unfairness of the adversarial malpractice system, amongst other factors.

Torn between the two sets of relevant and significant values, you are, as they say, on the horns of a dilemma. This is the nature of an ethical problem: it is the situation a person is in when forced to choose between two (or more) options, which have three characteristics:

(1) *Individually Convicting*: Each option has significant factors and/or reasonable arguments that make it morally appealing to you. Note: the truly difficult ethical choices are those between one good and another good, not between good and evil. The truly serious ethical questions have the form, "Of the two options, which good is better?"

(2) *Mutually Exclusive*: It is either one or the other. That does not mean that ethical problems can not be resolved by a compromise between the opposing options. Many are. But, the most difficult require us to choose one at the expense of rejecting the other. We either tell the parents, or we don't. We either intubate the 600 gram infant, or we don't. We either warn the HIV+ patient's sexual partner, or we don't. That's why ethical choices hurt so much: in order to achieve one good, we have to sacrifice another.

(3) *Jointly Demanding*: It has got to be one or the other. We must decide in two senses of the term. First, we are on the spot; it is up to us to decide. And, second, what we do will be decisive. Our action, one way or the other is determinative. The imperative nature of being in a dilemma means finally that even deciding *not* to decide is a decision, a decisive factor.

Given the importance of coming up with the best possible answers to these most serious dilemmas, we now need to examine how traditionally we have tried to formulate functional and defensible answers.

WHAT IS AN ETHICAL ANSWER?

Remember the nature of an ethical problem. It is when we find ourselves, literally, *in suspense* — suspended between individually appealing, mutually exclusive options, forcing us to decide. This produces literally, a "dis-ease". What is the treatment for this condition of ethical vertigo? Forced to take a stand, we must find a solid ground to stand on.

Grounding our judgement, which is to say grounding ourselves, is what gives us the necessary security, the *justifiable* security, to be able to act with confidence. For serious persons, ethical responsibilities are too heavy, too awesome to be handled with arbitrary, capricious or merely personal assertiveness. It is ironic how often people will say, without much reflection, that ethics is "just a matter of opinion", not realizing that in real situations serious persons take the differences between ethical options as anything but a mere matter of opinion.

No, persons really caught by an ethical dilemma do not trivialize the issue by acting as if the choices did not really make a difference, a moral difference, and that their responsibility was only to come up with an answer, any answer. Quite the opposite. If ethical persons have a fault, it is usually an excess of commitment, of conviction, of ultimate seriousness. Why? Because the responsibilities we bear for our patients, colleagues, families and communities are so significant, and the consequences of our judgements so serious, that we must justify the choices we make. Therefore, ethical judges seek to ground their individual judgements on some guiding and ordering structure, some authority-giving force.

HOW DO WE GROUND ETHICAL JUDGEMENTS?

There is a wide variety of answers to this question. But, there are three basic types of moves that persons make when they try to ground their individual judgements: principlist, contractualist, and consequentialist. While we discuss these three types, you might take your own ethical pulse, and check on which of these moves is (or are) expressive of your own decision-making process.

Principlist

This type of person looks for an absolute "truth" to ground our relative judgement, a universal rule to ground our individual actions. Figuratively, they "look up" to find some abiding higher principle, or a higher being, who defines the enduring structure of right and wrong. Examples would be in the form of ethical commandments, such as "Thou shalt not kill", or "Always tell the truth", or "Respect other's autonomy".

A "categorical imperative" is the way the 18th century philosopher Immanuel Kant described the ethical (and, one is tempted to add, the psychological) force of such principles.[4] They are "categorical" in the sense of not being contingent on anything else in a situation, and therefore not allowing any exceptions. For the principlist, the ethical person must obey the demands of the principle, regardless of circumstances or consequences. You must, for example, always tell the truth, even if it results in a danger of harm for yourself or others. Often this attitude is called "deontological" after the Greek word for duty, "deontos". But, the term "principlism" catches its spirit better, as expressed by a person insisting that she has to do something , and has to do it come-what-may, because, "It's a matter of principle!"

Which Principles Come First?

On the face of it, that question seems a bit peculiar. "Principles", by definition, are those elements of a system that come first. For principlists, they are precisely the determinative ground of all subsequent judgements and actions. But, different persons come to take different values as their principles. Which, then, have traditionally been the principles chosen most frequently by persons practicing medical ethics?

The answer has been given with striking uniformity over the last 15 years. This is due to the remarkable dominance of one basic introductory book, *Principles of Biomedical Ethics*, by Tom L. Beauchamp and James F. Childress.[5] First published in 1979, this quasi-Talmudic text presents four values as the prevalent determinative principles in biomedical ethics: respect for autonomy, beneficence, nonmaleficence, and justice. Since then, it seems as if virtually every other bioethical article has begun by ringing these four chimes. As they are so familiar, and so readily available in full detail in that classic text, let me here just briefly outline the essential content of each.*

Autonomy

Literally meaning "self-ruling" or "self-legislating", the principle of autonomy asserts the claim that each person has the right to make his or her own decisions, in his or her own way, based on his or her own values. Why such independence, such unilateral authority? Because each person is regarded as fundamentally "individual", a separate and distinct entity. Therefore, true respect for other persons requires us to respect assertions of their individuality, which they do by choosing how to live their own lives.

We need to underscore the principlist's application of the term "right" to autonomy. The nature of the individual makes autonomy a "right", a justifiably enforceable demand that creates for others an ethical duty that must be respected. For children, of course, there are serious questions about how individual they are, and hence, how "rightful" they should be considered. As mentioned, in Chapter 5 we shall attempt to custom-tailor this principle to fit the distinct reality of ethical relations with children.

Beneficence

This principle combines the spirit of "benevolence", of wishing well for others, with the practical obligation to use all one's knowledge and skill to make those good wishes come true. For the principled caregiver, beneficence expresses the categorical commitment to doing whatever you judge will best serve the best interests of the person in your care. Others' competing interests and your own conflicting interests must be excluded. Fulfillment of this ideal requires an exclusive and altruistic dedication to the other person, which Veatch has called "The core of professional physician ethics".[6] Its classic expression is found in that defining source of biomedical principles, the Oath of Hippocrates, "I will use treatment to help the sick according to my ability and judgement."

*In Chapter 5 on "Truthtelling", the two major principles, autonomy and beneficence, will be given close attention, and will set the parameters for shaping our practice regarding how much "heavy truth" we should place on a child.

Nonmaleficence

The line just quoted from the Oath continues, "but I will never use it to injure or wrong them." This is nonmaleficence: the principle of not-doing-harm to others. A loose Latin translation of a line from another part of the Hippocratic Corpus gives us what is often cited as the "first" principle of medicine: *Primum Non Nocere*, or "Above all do no harm". Much effort has been expended by thoughtful theoreticians, such as Beauchamp and Childress, explaining how these two principles are related, yet distinct. For our practical purposes, we may regard them as the two sides of the basic therapeutic commitment to serving the persons in your care: by maximizing the good done for them, and minimizing the harm done to them. One must provide the most helpful therapy, say for an osteosarcoma, but also reduce as much as possible any iatrogenic suffering as from amputation. Beneficence and nonmaleficence combine to dictate our duty to help the most and harm the least.*

Justice

The principle of justice expresses the binding sense of fairness in human relations. It has two major theoretical forms (which may in some situations conflict). The first, "retributive justice", mandates returning good for good (e.g., compensation for service, or rewards for achievement) and justifies returning bad for bad (e.g., punishment for crimes, or censure for misbehavior). The second, "distributive justice" expresses the sense of social equity in how we should order the distribution of the resources in a community. Again, we have literally thousands of years of attempts to delineate how to put this principle into practice. Perhaps the most classic summary formulation has been "From each according to ability; to each according to need."**

Let us just briefly illustrate the issues by asking whether pediatric practitioners would be justified in caring differently for two teenage HIV^+ patients, because one became infected by contaminated factor VIII for his hemophilia, and the other became infected by sharing his intravenous drug equipment? Or, an even more pervasive question of justice, should the amount of health care a child receives depend on the amount of payment his parent(s) can make?

We can distinguish between two types of principlists: the *rightful* principlists and the *virtuous* principlists. The rightful principlists appeal, not surprisingly, to "rights" as the ordering and empowering license for ethical actions. Acutely aware of the interpersonal nature of ethical action, they are ordered by the force of rights, of the justifiable demands that we make on others, and that others make on us. The rightful (or righteous?) principlist might insist that every person has a right to full and equal health care, or a right to be told the truth, or a right to confidentiality, and so forth. Each "right" becomes a command, a categorical command, that entails a duty to be fulfilled.

The other major adherents of principlism are the "virtuous principlists". They have the same rhythms and often end up in the same place as the rightful principlists, but they start

*A good example of how this should become operational will be found in Chapter 11 on the ethical management of pediatric pain.

**How social policy needs to consider such formulations is examined in Chapter 14, "Pediatric Practice, Social Responsibility and Physician Advocacy".

out from a different point. Their determinative authority comes from a sense of the moral virtues, regarded as innate standards that guide (or should) an individual's thoughts and actions. Aristotle's *Nichomachean Ethics*, as in part a primer for practical wisdom, analyzes and inculcates the moral virtues. What are the true virtues? Again we have centuries, indeed millennia, of debate. Certainly the virtues, taken by some as self-evident principles of behavior vested in the conscience of the moral individual, would include the following: *integrity*, acting in accord with one's centering values; *compassion*, sympathetic feeling producing commitment to others; *courage*, the willingness to maintain the right course despite fear or risk; *honesty*, the spirit of full and open communication with the other; and *loyalty*, the commitment to support those to whom we are bound.

To compare the two forms of principlism, consider our continuing dilemma. A rightful principlist might well ground telling the parents of the injured child on her sense of their right to know, therefore entailing a duty for her to fully inform them. The virtuous principlist might reach the same conclusion, but, his motivating force would be the virtuous spirit within demanding that he live up to the moral norm of honesty.

But, we should not make this seem like a too easy way to produce one-sided answers. For, it would also be an appeal to principlism if the pediatrician invoked the principle of promise-keeping as binding her to protect her colleague. And for the virtuous person, acting in the spirit of loyalty to colleagues might ground a refusal to reveal a harmful error. Principlism gives its adherents a way of guiding and grounding their judgements. But, it does not provide any specific set of ethical principles, nor any universal agreement on how to prioritize when principles conflict.

Contractualists

"Back to the future" might be the motto of the contractualist. To find what role they should play in shaping the future, they look to the past. For the contractualist perspective, we see the determinative structuring of the role we are now called to play in the obligations we assumed in the past.

Like the principlist, there is a categorical and unconditional nature to the determinative force in their ethical decision-making. But, unlike the principlists, there is usually an historical event or framework that has pre-emptively limited the ethically acceptable options in the present. Sexually, a contractualist would reject an affair because of the marriage vows. Scholastically, they would refuse to cheat on an exam because of having signed the Honor Code Pledge. Medically, they often take their stand on "the Oath" either by having made an *explicit* promise by reciting the Hippocratic Oath at graduation from medical school, or by having made an *implicit* commitment by accepting the traditional normative standards of their professional role.

Not too many years ago, when AIDS first surfaced, there was a collateral epidemic of ethical debate over the question of whether physicians were obligated to put themselves at risk to treat HIV^+ patients. Contractualists were split. The "explicit" contractualists argued that when they began their professional career (B.A., or Before AIDS) they never made a specific, informed agreement to treat HIV^+ patients; therefore, they now could choose not to. The "implicit" contractualists contended, on the other hand, that the altruistic tradition of medicine has always required a willingness to sacrifice yourself, even to put yourself in harm's way if necessary, in order to serve those in your care. Therefore, while the details of the obligation may change, the baseline contract, (or covenant), is binding and has pervasive authority.

For the contractualist, the individual finds the answers to specific ethical choices by analyzing the roles you have committed yourself to, for example, wife or husband, father or mother, physician or nurse, etc. The directive rubric? "Role Determines Rules". Ethically, one must fulfill the role you have contracted for. Each such role comes with a set of more or less explicit rules. Therefore, the decision-making process in any particular situation is, in effect, to study the *role-book* till you find the standards that predetermine the choices of the responsible, i.e., ethical, person.

Consider the example of whether to breach confidentiality for a 16-year-old who admits to serious drug use. The principlists would "look up" to find their ground for their answer in over-arching universals such as respect for autonomy or the right to privacy, or on virtues such as loyalty and fidelity. The contractualist, however, would "look back", either to an explicit promise made to this individual patient to keep and protect his confidences, or to the role-structuring tradition of medical practice that respects confidentiality as part of the implicit doctor-patient contract.

But, there is one other direction that many (indeed, probably most practitioners) would look to in order to find solid, justifiable answers: the future. Those who seek to ground their present answers in the future are called "consequentialists".

Consequentialists

What is the decision-making rhythm of consequentialists? It should be familiar for most of us. It is that of all clinical practitioners, in fact of all practical decision-makers. You have a newly diagnosed two-year-old with hepatoblastoma. First, you gather all possible courses of action. Surgery? Chemotherapy? Palliative care? Second, you examine all the most likely benefits and harms of each course. Third, you weigh these different packages in order to determine which will produce the most beneficial and least harmful future.

The practical decision-maker is like an author, imagining various ways to direct his or her characters, and calculating how future chains of consequences will be forged by these present choices. The ethical "author", or consequentialist, is the person who decides what ought to be done in the present by assessing which choice will produce the better package of consequences in the future.

What will the consequentialists do about the 16-year-old patient who has admitted drug use? First, there would be no principled or contractual restrictions on options. Any option that produces the maximum benefit would be permissible. Indeed, as maximizing beneficial consequences is the determinative moral imperative, whichever option promised to achieve the most beneficial future would be ethically obligatory. Therefore, the consequentialist would compare the benefits and harms of maintaining confidentiality: the adolescent feels secure and so cooperates more, more cooperation produces more guided protection, etc.; but, the physician cannot always be there, and keeping quiet may fail to alert other "life-guards", etc., On the other hand, "blowing the whistle" may get more help, more control and more protection, etc.; but, it might just drive the kid away from trusting any adult, and produce more drug abuse as a passive–aggressive or defensive reaction to a perceived betrayal, and so on, and on, and on.

The basic decision-making process for the consequentialist may be described in a quasi-mathematical formulation:

Step One: For Option A, add up all the possible benefits and possible harms, and factor the probability of each.

Step Two: Subtract the value of the harms from the value of the benefits to get the net value of Option A.

Step Three: Repeat for Option B (and Option C, etc.).

Step Four: Compare the Net Value of Option A versus the Net Value of Option B (and C, etc.).

Step Five: Whichever option has the better (or less bad) net value is the ethically appropriate/obligatory choice.

Consequentialists are allowed to be much more independent, much more empowered than principlists or contractualists to act on the basis of their own judgement. For example, neither a principle such as autonomy, nor a contract, whether explicit or implicit, would preclude breaking confidentiality, if the consequentialist judged that action would produce better consequences. One could break promises, or lie, or choose any other action, so long as it could justifiably be claimed that your intention was to produce the greatest possible good, and that your calculation had fairly demonstrated that the course you chose would most likely achieve that end.

Joseph Fletcher, the founding person for a consequentialist approach to medical ethics, cited as the model for one of his major books a St. Louis cab driver, who, after explaining that he was going to vote Democratic although he and his family had been life-long Republicans, said, "[T]here are times when a man has to push his principles aside and do the right thing."[7]

However, given the dangers of this self-appointed authority to act on one's own individual calculations, and of this self-licensed liberty to override principles and contracts, there clearly is an imperative need to make such calculations with great discipline. Nowhere is the need greater for employing and enforcing the normative standards of the good judge, than when the judge is a consequentialist, and the judgements will have irreversible consequences for the critical needs and interests of patients and families in our care.

TESTING YOUR DECISIONING

Ultimately, every true professional must be self-policing. Our ethical responsibility is to check and challenge ourselves as though we were our own strongest opponents. Even more, our obligation is to never lose the fear that we may turn out to be the worst enemy for those we most care about. Feeling that we are doing good and intending to do good are not enough. All too often they are precisely the most dangerously deceptive disguises, concealing from others and from ourselves how harmful our "good actions" may be.

How do we police ourselves, and others? Not by tongue-wrestling over which principles or other value-claims should prevail. We discipline ourselves and others in our ethical decision-making the same way we do in our clinical decision-making. We uphold and administer the standards of the professional role. Recall the section on the good judge to check on those standards: knowledgeable, impartial, systemic, decisive, corrigible and empathetic.

But, in addition we need to use a set of procedural checks. These should serve to constantly challenge how well we are managing the complex range of facts and values necessary for truly realistic, responsive and responsible decision-making. We should regard these as a set of chronic questions designed to express and exacerbate what should be every ethical judge's inalienable sense of self-doubt.

(1) *How Clear*? Have I actually seen each factor as it is, and have I incorporated it into my system without distortions?

(2) *How Consistent*? Have I used key concepts consistently? Have I respected terms or values not only when they would serve my purposes or interests, but also when they would inhibit them?

(3) *How Coherent*? Have I checked that all of the clear and consistent parts in my judgement truly fit together without contradictions or gaps? Like a good geometric proof, do I have a solid ground and an orderly sequence of steps building from that ground to a rationally connected conclusion?

(4) *How Comprehensive*? Have I taken into account all relevant factors? Or, have I included only the preferred elements and edited out the confounding views and factors?

(5) *How Conclusive*? Have I openly recognized and honestly refuted all countervailing views and arguments? Have I fairly won the right to claim that my conclusion is conclusive?

What do all these challenges require? That we recognize how the high seriousness of ethical judgement in medical practice demands that we apply the highest standards of disciplined judgement. "From Principles to Practice" is the sub-title of this book. That has two senses: first, it points to the need to ground our individual choices and actions in pediatric practice on a structure of substantive values; and, second, it underscores the ethical obligation we have as responsible practitioners and persons to put principles into the process by which we make our judgements about ethical issues. The purpose of this chapter especially, and of this whole volume is to foster our understanding of the importance, and rewards, of practicing with such principles.

References

1. Brody, H. (1976). *Ethical Decisions in Medicine*, Boston: Little Brown, p. 19.
2. Bridge, P. and Bridge, M. (1981). The Brief Life and Death of Christopher Bridge. *Hastings Report*, **11**(6), p. 19.

3. Eliot, G. (1860). *The Mill on the Floss*, New York: Penguin, (1979), p. 628.
4. Kant, I. (1984). *Groundwork of the Metaphysic of Morals*, trans, H. J. Paton, New York, Harper & Row.
5. Beauchamp, T. L. and Childress, J. F. (1989). *Principles of Biomedical Ethics*, New York: Oxford University Press.
6. Veatch, R. M. (1981). *A Theory of Medical Ethics*, New York: Basic Books, p. 22.
7. Fletcher, J. (1966). *Situation Ethics*, Philadelphia: Westminster Press, p. 13.

2 A Time to Die: Ethical, Legal and Professional Grounds for Judgement

Robert C. Cassidy

Schneider Children's Hospital, Long Island Jewish Medical Center, 269-01 76th Avenue, New Hyde Park, New York 11040, USA

FOREWORD

In 1976 two highly qualified and experienced pediatricians participated in a symposium in Montreal, Dr. John Lorber from England, and Dr. John Freeman from Johns Hopkins. Both were particularly distinguished for their care of newborn children with spina bifida and myelomeningocele.

However, their choices of treatment (or non-treatment) for the life-threatening lesion were radically different. Dr. Freeman withheld potentially life-saving surgery from only 5% of his patients, while Dr. Lorber, with similar cases, withheld such treatment from 75% of his patients.

Commenting on this striking difference, Dr. Freeman expressed his painful perplexity:

> With equal conscience and good will, Dr. Lorber and I treat widely different numbers of patients. I fail to believe that either of us is unethical. And yet, we both can't be right — or can we?[1]

INTRODUCTION

With the poignance felt only by those whose decisions have real life-or-death consequences, Dr. Freeman poses the most serious and difficult challenge for persons who would be ethical: how can we know which answer is right?

The problem is not produced, as some would have it, because there are no answers. Rather the problem is that there are too many answers: too many opposing views and values, and too many diverse judges each demanding that their "right" should rule.

As a philospher once said, The Book of Life comes with a multiple-choice test — but, without an answer sheet in the back of the book. Absent an answer sheet, absent clear and universal and absolute answers, individuals are obliged to choose the good. And ethical individuals are obliged to choose the good in the best way possible.

The question this chapter deals with is Dr. Freeman's question: When is choosing death for a child justified? That's what ethics is all about. As we discussed in Chapter 1, ethics is the art of justifying choices about power. As with any art, some are better at it than others: more focused, more committed, more disciplined, more informed, and more reflective. And, as with any art, most become better by working longer and harder, and in the company of other skilled practitioners.

The past 20 years have produced a remarkable concentration of disciplined attention to the question of when we should forego life-extending treatment. In particular, the most distinguished medical and legal and ethical organizations have labored to bring forth their best judgement, in order to help individual practitioners' make their judgements better. The purpose of this chapter is to draw us into that good company of serious judges.

We shall begin with the 1982 "Baby Doe Case", concentrating on the values and arguments that generated the Federal regulations. Then we shall explore the thinking of the pediatric profession, as expressed through the two major position papers of the American Academy of Pediatrics. We shall conclude by examining the work of two task forces composed of ethical, legal and medical experts: the 1983 Report of The President's Commission for the Study of Ethical Problems in Medicine and Biomedical and Behavioral Research; and the ethical guidelines for deciding about "imperiled newborns" developed at The Hastings Center, for 25 years the leading force in the United States for transforming bioethical controversy into disciplined judgements.

Throughout this tour of the greater bioethical community, we shall be particularly seeking guidance on two critical aspects of decisions about foregoing life-extending treatment: First, which children should be allowed to die? and Second, how much discretion should individuals, either parents or physicians, be allowed to have in answering the first question?

Finally, challenging all judgements, theirs and ours, is one fundamental question: what makes one judgement, or one judge, better than another?

NORMATIVE VIEWS

Before we begin our historical tour, however, we should plot three normative views that ground many of the specific positions. As Paul Ramsey would have insisted, "There are no ethics without ultimates." Much of the dynamics of the debate over foregoing treatment will be shaped by how the different judges balance (or are balanced by) three ethical ultimates: sanctity of life, quality of life, and social utility.

1. Sanctity of Life: A Categorical Imperative

According to this view, each human life is *inalienably* good, *equally* good, *intrinsically* good, and *pre-eminently* good. "Inalienably" good means that it has enduring value regardless of quality, condition, capacity, or any other characteristic. The presence or absence of any characteristic, mental or physical, does not affect the value of the life nor, consequently, the duty to treat. Therefore, a child could not be denied life-saving treatment because of any degree of mental or physical disability, nor because of the presence of overwhelming suffering.

Second, each living person is of equal value. As individuating characteristics do not count, no person could be worth more, or less, than any other. A child with a high I.Q. is worth no more. A child with quadriplegia is worth no less. As, Dr. C. Everett Koop has written in an article provocatively titled, "The Slide to Auschwitz", "Each newborn infant, perfect or deformed, is a human being, with unique preciousness."[2]

Third, the value of each child is intrinsic, which means its value is not dependent on anything outside itself. Its value is not dependent on fulfilling its family's desires or serving its society's interests, or satisfying any other purpose. Human persons are valuable in and of themselves, and not because they are judged useful to, or valued by, others.

Finally, for these "vitalists", as they are called, life is the pre-eminent good. There is no greater good for which it could justifiably be sacrificed. Its claims on us may never be ethically evaded or compromised. For the religious vitalists, the duty to respect the sanctity of life comes from the absolute commandment of the ultimate lord of every human life, and every human choice. For all vitalists, each human life confronts us as a categorical imperative: an unqualified good demanding unconditional care.

2. Quality of Life: A Personal Judgement

The slogan "quality of life" has come to be used (and abused) to describe those who believe that it is the qualities of a life that make it valuable; that some individuals have significantly less of some qualities; and, that some degree of qualitative deficit justifies foregoing life-extending treatment. In sum, quality of life may determine quantity of care.

Rejecting vitalism's quasi-mystical devotion to "life", such "personalists" view the value of an individual's life as a matter of judgement about how much value this life has *for that individual*. The nature of this value is predominantly experiential, comprising such positive aspects as enjoyment, achievement, love, comfort, security and independence — and such negative aspects as pain, fear, anxiety, stress, frustration, vulnerability, loneliness and dependency.

A quality of life calculus prognostically weighs the degree of capacity for positive experiences and subtracts the degree of actual or anticipated negative experiences, both the presence of harms and the absence of benefits. Then, if the balance of burdens over benefits becomes, in the mind of the judge, significantly disproportionate, the ethically responsible guardian of the person's welfare may act to protect that person from the harm of further life.

The ethical commitment for the personalist should be to the person, not to life, *per se*. Life, if good for the person, is good. But, life is not always good. Neither is life always better than death. When life for a person in our care is judged a fate worse than death, then death may be, indeed *should* be, the treatment of choice, of rational and humane choice.

3. Social Utility: The Greatest Good

For vitalists, life is always good. For personalists, death is sometimes better, or less bad. But, both vitalists and personalists base their judgements exclusively on what they judge good for the individual person.

By contrast, another ethical perspective, traditionally called social utilitarianism, regards this individualistic limit of concern as unrealistic and irresponsible. Persons are not just individuals. What they are and what is required for their care impact substantively on others. The overwhelmingly devastating burdens of the lives of severely damaged children fall not only on them but on their families — and on society.

The vision of social utilitarians encompasses the whole range of benefits and burdens produced by a life. Valuing the lives of all, they will refuse to allow the extreme needs of one to mute the appeal of the competing needs of others. Rather, in the classic social utilitarian calculus, they will insist on the ethical duty to weigh and balance the interests of all, and then act so as to produce "The greatest good of the greatest number."

Two consequences follow from such a commitment to weighing the full range of consequences. First, to some degree decisions to forego life-sustaining treatment may be tilted by the degree of burdening and suffering imposed by someone's life on his or her family. Second, the cost to society will be granted a hearing in the social utilitarian's court. Specifically, concerns about how best to allocate scarce resources may justify withholding marginally beneficial and economically voracious life-sustaining treatment from some in order to produce a greater amount of good for others.

However, opponents of social utilitarianism often raise the specter of the slippery slope. This argument warns us to beware of the future consequences of the precedents we create in individual cases. Sacrificing even one person, no matter how devastated the conditions and costly the care, may set us on an inevitable slide towards uncontrolled license in many other cases. Hence, the ominous warning about the inertial dangers of using some for the sake of others in Dr. Koop's title, "The Slide to Auschwitz."

Now, with this metaphysical map in hand, it is time to begin our exploration of the ethical, legal and professional foundations for pediatric euthanasia judgements.

THE BABY DOE CASE AND THE ROLE OF REGULATIONS

On Friday, April 9, 1982, a baby boy with Down's syndrome was born in Bloomington, Indiana. Two weeks later he was dead. His real name has never become public. But, as "Baby Doe", his brief life became the focus for governmental attempts to set public limits on previously private decisions to choose death for children. As a New York Times editorial declared, "The death of Infant Doe is not a private matter."[3]

Unfortunately, the substantive ethical and social significance of this event has mostly been overlooked in the midst of the polemical battles over the tone and tactics of the Federal response. Despite the political acrimony and rhetorical excesses on both sides of the controversy, this case remains significant as the first attempt by the Federal government to answer the questions of what gives commanding value to an infant's life, and what conditions if any, could justify deciding to forego life-extending care.

For our purpose of analyzing possible grounds for individual decision-making, we shall ignore the smoke-screen of politicized controversy and examine the normative and procedural standards generated by both sides. We may be surprised to realize how substantive and determinative these standards have become. In anticipation, let us note the major components of the government's position: first, decisions to forego care are permitted under some circumstances; second, despite various denials, the circumstances are quality-of-life factors; and third, substantial discretion is permitted to caregivers, primarily to physicians, in making such life-ending choices.

A Brief History

Baby Doe was born with Down's syndrome, the most common physical malformation and mental retardation syndrome, occurring in 1 in 700 to 1 in 1000 newborns.[4] In addition to an anticipated (but undetermined) degree of mental retardation, Baby Doe also had esophageal atresia with associated tracheoesophageal fistula. As a result, he needed a surgical repair of his digestive tract (or some alternative procedure) in order to be fed effectively.

However, the parents refused to give consent to surgery for their baby. Despite legal appeals from some of Baby Doe's caregivers, the local and state courts refused to intervene, implicitly upholding the right of the parents to choose. The baby died before an emergency appeal could be heard by the United States Supreme Court.

Just two weeks later, then President Reagan sent a personal letter to the Secretary of Health and Human Services declaring his commitment to protecting handicapped newborns such as Baby Doe:

> Our nation's commitment to equal protection of the law will have little meaning if we deny such protection to those who have not been blessed with the same physical and mental gifts we too often take for granted.[5]

Placing this case under the rubric of discrimination against the handicapped, President Reagan invoked Section 504 of the Rehabilitation Act of 1973 as the license for Federal intervention.[6]

What followed was a series of confrontational moves and counter-moves by Federal agencies, medical and hospital organizations, Federal courts, and ultimately, the United States Congress, which produced The Child Abuse Prevention and Treatment Act Amendments of 1984[7], which, with accompanying interpretive rules published by The Department of Health and Human Services,[8] became the final form of the government's regulatory vision.

We should note that these regulations were not a unilateral declaration by the government. Rather, they were the product of extensive negotiations with professional organizations, leading advocacy groups, and the members of Congress drafting the Child Abuse Amendments bill. These included the American Hospital Association, The American Academy of Pediatrics, The American Nurses Association, The National Association of Children's Hospitals and Related Institutions, The American College of Obstetricians and Gynecologists, The American College of Physicians and The Association for Retarded Citizens of the United States.

The Regulations basically promulgated three moves designed to protect infants from harm. First, they redefined "medical neglect" to specifically include infants. Second, they redefined what it means to withhold "medically indicated treatment". And, third, they described three medical conditions that would justify withholding otherwise required treatment. Let us examine the meaning of, and rationale for, each of these regulatory moves.

1. "Medical Neglect"

For the Government, Baby Doe's case demonstrated that some infants had suffered from a *de facto* suspension of the usual measures designed to protect children against neglect. Therefore, they redefined "medical neglect" specifically to include "withholding of medically indicated treatment *from a disabled infant* with a life-threatening condition."[9]

As the ultimate guardian and guarantor of the welfare of all citizens, the government was outraged by the failure to protect the life of Baby Doe. As *parens patriae* (literally, "parent of the country"), they asserted their right and duty to protect the best interests of their most vulnerable "children". Further, they insisted that the duty to protect from harm encompasses intervening, if necessary, to protect children from their purported care providers, whether medical or parental.

Such a duty to protect children from harm has traditionally been required of, and exercised by all responsible caregivers. Included in this is the duty to oppose anyone who does not exercise a minimum degree of care in supplying a child with (among other needs) adequate medical or surgical care. Pediatricians, as those professionals most committed to child-advocacy, should be especially diligent and responsible in fulfilling this duty.[10]

Building on this basic obligation, the government asserts that withholding medically indicated treatment from newborns is not exempt from the duty to provide care and prevent harm. Failure to provide medically beneficial treatment is harmful for children of any age.

2. "Medically indicated Treatment"

The focal concern is a child with life-threatening conditions. Quite simply, only treatment which can reverse those threats, all those threats, will benefit the child. And for the government only such treatment is mandatory. Remember Baby Doe: the child's only life-threatening condition was the fistula. Surgery had a reasonably good chance of correcting that condition, thereby saving the child's life. That is the paradigm of medically beneficial, and thus, mandatory treatment. If, however, the life-threatening conditions cannot be removed, then further treatment may be regarded as not beneficial, and so not mandatory.

We should also note that the government has not imposed a demand for any specific treatments on physicians. Quite the contrary! With surprising emphasis, the statute stipulates that the attending physician's "reasonable medical judgement" determines what is medically beneficial. Even nutrition, hydration and medication, which some have read as always required, are only required when "appropriate", which again is left to reasonable medical judgement.

Finally, the government explicitly excludes any social utilitarian considerations of the burdens on others, whether on society or on families. The child's needs and welfare must be the exclusive concern.

3. Exceptions

Any of three medical conditions justify withholding treatment.

(1) The infant is chronically and irreversibly comatose;

(2) The provision of such treatment would merely prolong dying, not be effective in ameliorating or correcting all of the infant's life-threatening conditions, or otherwise be futile in terms of the survival of the infant; or

(3) The provision of such treatment would be virtually futile in terms of the survival of the infant, and the treatment itself under such circumstances would be inhumane.[11]

Now, let us examine each of these in some detail. Remarkably, each of these exceptions invokes a quite distinct ethical license for non-treatment.

Let us take the second one first, as it is the logical complement to only requiring "beneficial" treatment. Ineffective treatment is not required. Specifically, if treatment cannot save the child's life then it is not beneficial and, therefore, is not required.

"Futile" treatment is specifically exempted. But, more than that. Treatment which would "merely prolong dying" is also exempted. Now, that is a substantial extension of discretion, for it means that even if treatment could effectively lengthen a child's life, it still could be withheld if it would not completely correct the life-threatening condition. In other words, a limited amount of life is judged such a limited benefit as to not be required. In effect, the standard is that if a child is inescapably going to die soon, then sooner is not substantively worse for the child than later.

When we also note that there is no longer (as in earlier versions) any restrictive definition of "dying" or "terminal", we must recognize that this standard could well encompass decisions to deny weeks or even months of life to a child. The Child Abuse Amendments April 15, 1985 Final Rule eliminated the requirement that the infant's death be "imminent" in order to justify foregoing treatment. No time limit is fixed. No definition of "dying" is pronounced. As a result, the Final Rule authorizes a broad latitude for discretionary judgement by attending physicians about when an infant's quantity of life should determine the quantity of treatment.

It is within the range of reasonable medical judgement to decide that a 22 week, 450 gram premature infant (who might live a few hours or days) is dying — or that a trisomy-13 or trisomy-18 infant (who might live a few months) is dying, — but, might it also be within the range of reasonable judgement to hold that a child with Lesch–Nyhan syndrome or a Tay–Sachs disease (who might live a few years) is dying? The point is that *whether* a child should be regarded as dying is a matter of judgement; and, note please, the regulations license a remarkable degree of latitude for physicians to make such judgements. This clearly is not the monolatrous vitalism that some critics have accused the government of imposing.

Now, consider the first exception: "The infant is chronically and irreversibly comatose." Quite simply, despite all denials, this is a "quality-of-life" judgement. A child with no chance of ever having a conscious life is judged to not have a life that must be saved. Though not stated openly, the reasoning is clear. The quality of the life is so negligible that there is no real benefit to the child in having the life extended, nor real harm to the child in having the life ended.

But, there is still a real line drawn here. Only total absence of consciousness justifies withholding treatment. This allows the government to take a stand on an ostensibly objective, and therefore, functionally more defensible line. Irreversible coma is a matter of medical judgement, which can be policed by medical procedures in accordance with medical standards. Requiring treatment for all children with any degree of consciousness, no matter how minimal, sets a quite rigid restraint on subjective judgements of "a life worth living," and may impede the slide down the slippery slope.

The third exception is in many ways the most surprising, for it authorizes caregivers to make decisions based on their judgements of the harms and benefits of treatment. If life-saving treatment is judged "virtually futile" (i.e., minimally beneficial), and treatment is judged "inhumane" (i.e., significantly harmful), then treatment may be foregone.

The ethical license involved here is derived from the Principle of Proportionality: a rational and humane moral calculus of the benefits and burdens of treatment. We are authorized to judge that for some children the chance of benefit (cure or survival) is so small, and the agonizing burdens of treatment are so great (pain or suffering) that guardians may choose to act to protect the child from further treatment, and further life.

In summary, the core of the government's position (reached, as we noted, in conjunction with the major professional organizations dedicated to caring for children) establishes rules for reasonable medical judgement of the condition of newborn infants, and reasonable ethical judgement of their best interests to serve as grounds for foregoing life-extending care. Responsible judges, i.e., pediatricians, are authorized to be discriminating. And when life-extending treatment will not benefit a child, or will clearly produce more harm than benefit, then responsible medical guardians may forego extending the life of that child.

THE ACADEMY AS AUTHORITY

Since the very beginning, membership in the profession of medicine has meant subscribing to a set of standards. Such "codes", whether the Oath of Hippocrates or The American Medical Association's "Principles of Medical Ethics" (whose formulation in 1847 was the gestational work of the embryonic guild), have defined the standards of the profession and delimited the behavior of the professionals. In fact, having such an explicit authoritative code is a defining mark of a profession.[12]

Since its founding in 1930 in the United States, the American Academy of Pediatrics (AAP) has served as the authoritative voice of the pediatric profession. If we are to find a guiding and grounding voice from within the profession, surely the pronouncements of the AAP must receive close attention. In 1983, stimulated (or provoked) by the Federal intervention in the Baby Doe case, the AAP did formulate and publish an official policy on the "Treatment of Critically Ill Newborns".[13] Perhaps because of the limitations of that first attempt, in 1994 a second set of "Guidelines on Forgoing Life-Sustaining Medical Treatment" was published.[14] We shall analyze both these efforts to ground and guide pediatric decision-making. We shall conclude this section with a brief account of the parallel position of the American Medical Association.

1983 AAP Policy: "On Treatment of Critically Ill Newborns"

In order to be effective, any professional policy must have three components: *grounding principles* to frame individual decisions; *clear criteria* for putting those principles into practice; and an *operational process* for employing the criteria. Unfortunately, the original one and one-half page *Guidelines* produced by the AAP in 1983 offers only glimpses of such an effective instrument. After mention of the range of malformations from anencephalics through Down's syndrome children, they acknowledge their inability to:

> identify a consensus on which infants or children within this broad range should be treated.[14]

Therefore, while quickly rejecting a categorical commitment to treat all, as not serving the interests of some, they decline to offer any criteria for selection. As they admit:

> The range of complexity in these conditions make it impossible to define clinical criteria for withholding treatment.[15]

Despite this lack of clinical consensus, the policy does claim "consensus on some ethical principles." However, they offer only one principle: "The pediatrician's primary obligation is to the child." We are advised that when the child's interests are clear, they should not be sacrificed to competing family interests. However, if the child's interests are less clear (for example, when his or her life will be dominated by suffering), then the concerns of the family "may play a larger role". But, since they themselves have recognized how the complexity of these cases and the variety of the judges preclude clarity, it is hard to derive any functional guidance from such "principles".

Their only other "principle" is the insistence that such profound judgements should be "made carefully and in an informed manner."[16] Although this also seems to offer little useful guidance, it does ground the one contentful component of the AAP policy: a procedural proposal for Infant Bioethical Review Committees. The sensitivity and complexity of these decisions preclude having a single physician as the sole judge, they conclude. Therefore, a committee process is recommended in the form of a group consultation with other individuals with complementary medical, ethical, and social expertise. To assure accountability, such a group should be constituted as a formal institutional entity. To avoid disrupting established responsibility, it should still only serve as a consultant to the pediatrician, who continues to act as the "primary physician".*

In summary, the Academy was attempting to avoid espousing either of the extremes of an undisciplined individualism, which might let viable infants die, or an insensitive legalism, which might insensitively sacrifice infants to ideology. But, absent definite principles and defined criteria, the Academy's espousal of committees as a responsible and responsive middle ground offers little substantive guidance for deciding about complex individual cases. It is perhaps more than coincidental that the next effort of the AAP does not even mention their own earlier effort.

* Chapter 4 in this volume presents a thorough history and critique of Pediatric Ethics Committees

1994 AAP Guidelines on Foregoing Life-Sustaining Medical Treatment

These "guidelines" present an excellent set of constructive principles and useful criteria for the decision-making process in pediatric care. Focused and detailed proposals are presented for dealing with the principal issues in balancing the roles of physicians, patients and their families. It could serve as an excellent guide to enlightened communications for all medical practice. However, as truly valuable as this may be, the 1994 "guidelines" still shy away from providing contentful guidelines for decisions to forego life-sustaining treatment.

What do they offer? First, a very important underwriting of the duty to respect the views of "child patients". More than just benign lip service, they require "careful, *explicit* attention to the wishes and feelings of children." This includes a strong endorsement of informing young children of their critical condition and of decisions to forego further treatment, and specific standards for responsibly assessing a child's decision-making capacity.

A second major position is their affirmation of the primacy of parents as the presumptive surrogates for children without capacity. Invoking the principle of respect for family automony, the academy insists that when patients are incapacitated, their families should be granted "wide discretion in making their own decisions" about foregoing treatment. Only when their wishes "clearly conflict" with the best interests of the child, should professionals oppose the family judgement.

Their third useful contribution is to endorse several consensus views on which treatments are optional. They include artificial nutrition and hydration in this category and they also agree that there is no substantive ethical or legal distinction between withholding and withdrawing treatment.

Finally, they approve the use of a "best interests" standard, and provide an extensive list of the specific benefits and burdens that should be assayed in this medical/moral calculus.

What, then is lacking? Two major elements. First, aside from one paragraph which recites the trinitarian refrain of *beneficence, nonmaleficence* and *autonomy*, there is no attempt to ground their stipulations on any systematic structure of critical reflection and principled judgement. Second, they carefully avoid giving any indication of where the lines should be drawn. No condition, no syndrome, and no case of any sort is offered to define and delimit the appropriate and inappropriate situations for foregoing life-extending treatment.

In sum, this second attempt is a much more serious offering of procedural guidelines, notable for recognizing the *prima facie* order of authority as patient first, parents second, and pediatricians third. But, the Academy still is unwilling or unable to provide substantive guidelines for those who must bear the responsibility of choosing to forego life-sustaining care.

1981 AMA Code of Medical Ethics

In 1981 the American Medical Association also issued an official pronouncement on the issue of euthanasia, including decisions for infants, which regrettably shares much the same values, and vagueness, as the AAP policy.[17] Foregoing life-extending treatment is approved as ethical in some circumstances, but no specific criteria are delineated in the one paragraph allocated to this issue. They express a primary commitment to life, even with handicaps; but, they draw the line at prolonging a life when it would be "inhumane and unconscionable".

As does the AAP, so the AMA declares that the "primary consideration should be the best interests of the patient, and not the avoidance of burdens to the family or society." In such decisions, the AMA does specifically endorse "Quality of Life" as a factor, a position which directly challenges the Federal rejection of such judgements. But, again no contentful criteria are proffered for judging the "best interests" of a child and we are left with a vague license to make discretionary judgements about life-prolonging treatments, but with no clear, structural guidance.

As an historical footnote, it is interesting to note a deletion. In the 1981 edition, the AMA explicitly identified the parents, not the physicians, as the most appropriate surrogates to decide about sustaining the life of a severely defective newborn. This empowering of parents was deleted from the 1992 edition.

THE BIOETHICAL CENTER: THE REPORT FROM HASTINGS

Ever since its founding in 1970, the Hastings Center has served as the mother house for the burgeoning profession of bioethics. Its *Report* has provided the leading forum for collegial exchange, and its educational programs have affected virtually all who practice as professional, or semi-professional, bioethicists.

In recent years, the Center has drawn together members from its professional staff and leaders from the international bioethical community to produce task force reports, which they modestly describe as frameworks of, and for, moral analysis.

In 1987, the Hastings Center produced "Imperiled Newborns", the report of its research project on the Care of Imperiled Newborns, directed by Arthur Caplan and composed of a score of distinguished bioethical experts.[20] They concentrate much of their attention on the question of how we should determine whether treatment or non-treatment is ethically right for a particular infant. However, such particular judgements can only be formulated, they insist, if we have established "reasonable standards of judgement".[21] Two standards of judgement set the framework for their analysis: sanctity of life and quality of life.

Sanctity of Life Standard

In the extreme form of "vitalism" (as described above), the Sanctity of Life Standard demands an "unqualitized" and, consequently, unqualified commitment of all care for all children. The value of each human life is absolute, and absolutely equal. Any consideration of what qualities it has, e.g., mental or physical capacities, is irrelevant (if not irreverent), and any restriction of the quantity of care because of the qualities of the life is an unjustifiable offense.

For the Task Force, however, such vitalism represents a blind respect for the principle of life, at the expense of a sensitive regard for the needs of the living. Forcing painful treatment on a dying infant is the paradigm of the insensitive and irresponsible impact of such an inhumane ideal on real human beings.

The Department of Health and Human Services in "Baby Doe Rules", are regarded as a milder variant of the Sanctity of Life Standard.

The Task Force views the Federal regulators as favoring a "non-discriminating" standard of judgement in order to defend a non-discriminatory policy. The intent of their "Medical Indications" Policy is to limit discretionary judgements by setting purportedly objective, factual, scientifically determined categories, and then to demand equal treatment for all in that category. Thus, the neurologically normal child, the Down's syndrome child, and a neurologically devastated child with only a flicker of painful consciousness are all in the same category: non-terminal, non-comatose patients. Any discriminating between them would be, for the government's policy, "discriminatory", and thus, categorically unfair.

A "Medical Benefits Standard" reinforces the Federal non-discriminatory standard. Physicians are enjoined not to ask whether a treatment will serve the person, but whether it will solve the problem. For example, a trisomy-13 child might go into pulmonary failure. The Medical Benefits Standard would only allow us to ask whether mechanical ventilation would help solve the respiratory dysfunction, but not to ask whether it would benefit the person to be kept alive longer.

The Task Force rejects such a rigid and myopic bio-medical standard of "benefit". Discrimination is wrong because it treats persons who are the same differently. But, a child with a truly devastating handicap truly is different from a normally endowed child. To blind ourselves to that reality is to abdicate from the role of responsive and responsible judges. Further, we must not compound that rigidity by refusing to acknowledge that a treatment could be medically "successful", but still humanly harmful. We must not allow fear of the abuse of judgement to paralyze and anesthetize the judges. Discriminating judgement, therefore, is not only ethically justifiable, but mandatory.

Quality of Life Standard

Discriminating between infants and consequently between giving or forgoing life-extending treatment does pose real dangers of abuse. The Task Force begins its analysis of the Quality of Life Standard it approves by eliminating the variants it rejects.

First, the positive and negative qualities to be weighed must only be those in and for the child. Allowing harms and benefits to family or to society to alter care of the infant is prohibited. Unfortunately, such a categorical exclusion is asserted, but not argued.

Second, the Task Force warns against projecting our own reasonably *un*handicapped lives as the standard of an "acceptable" quality of life for others. The Promethean capacity of the handicapped to fulfill and enjoy the opportunities of their own unique lives is legend. We are cautioned to keep the world safe for diversity.

Positively, then, what does the Task Force propose? In their words, it is a "Best Interest/Relational Potential" standard[22] which holds that infants should receive all life-sustaining treatment, except when (1) Terminal: the infant is dying, or (2) Futile: the treatment is medically contra-indicated, or (3) Harmful: more life would be worse than death. For this last category the paradigm would be a life of severe and intractable pain.

But, more than the absence of pain is necessary to give a life the quality which compels our care. Drawing on the proposal of Father Richard McCormick,[23] the Task Force proposes that the level of quality of life that obligates us to provide life-extending treatment is a life that has a "present capacity or future potential for human relationships".[24]

An infant who lacks all such capacity or potential for human interaction, the Task Force argues, "cannot be said to have interests" in being kept alive. Treatment for such a depersonalized being is not required, because treatment offers no personal benefit. But, neither is non-treatment required, because continued treatment, and life, impose no harm.

Note that this standard would authorize non-treatment for more children then the Federal category of "clinically and permanently unconscious". This class of the relationally handicapped, or, what we might call, the "permanently impersonal", would include those with some degree of consciousness, but with such profound retardation that there was no present or future capacity for consciousness of another person.

Great caution and patience are urged to be certain that an individual infant has no reasonable possibility of an interpersonal existence. Judging that a child is "permanently impersonal" is obviously extraordinarily difficult, especially given the infant's anomalous and mysteriously plastic capacity for neurological regeneration. But, when reasonable medical certainty is achieved, the Task Force believes a disciplined process of judgement operating in accordance with this Best Interests/Relational Potential Standard, would be ethically justified in deciding to withhold or withdraw life-sustaining care.

THE PRESIDENT'S COMMISSION

In 1979, the President's Commission for the Study of Ethical Problems in Medicine and Biomedical and Behavioral Research was constituted by an Act of Congress. The President's Commission produced an enormous body of published work, including major studies of *Making Health Care Decisions* in 1982[25] and *Deciding to Forego Life Sustaining Treatment* in 1983,[26] which were based on written papers and extensive oral presentations from all the major health care institutions and agencies, and from leading scholars from the medical, legal and ethical communities.

When they addressed the questions of deciding to forego life-sustaining treatment for infants and young children, they concentrated on two questions. First, What should be the standards *for* judging, i.e., how should we judge? and second, what should be the standards *of* judgement, i.e., what conditions should determine our judgements? Their special concern was to create structural answers to these two questions that would address the special problems and responsibilities of *surrogate* decision-makers, who must justify deciding about life-and-death for persons who cannot speak for themselves.

Surrogate decision-makers for adult incompetent patients usually invoke two standards to justify deciding for another person. The *Substituted Judgement Standard* claims that a surrogate can judge what a particular person would want in this situation because of knowledge of that person's basic values as expressed in either general statements (e.g.,

"Being able to work and live my own life is more important to me than anything.") or in specific statements about similar situations (e.g., "I'd never want to be tube fed like Dad was."). This might better be called the *Representative* Judgement Standard, in the sense that the surrogate's authority comes from being able to "re-present" the individual patient's views and values.

However, for persons who have not developed and expressed an individual value history, the Substituted Judgement Standard is inapplicable. Newborns and young children are such "anonymous persons." Therefore, since we are unable to claim to know what an individual "Baby Billy" or "Baby Mary" would want, the best we can do is to claim to know what best serves the interests of this sort of patient with this sort of condition.

This is called the *Best Interests Standard.* It asks, "What is reasonably certain most persons in this condition would want?" As applied to most pediatric decisions to forego life-extending care, the question becomes, "Under these conditions, is it reasonably certain that most children would not want their life extended?" As the Commission declares, when Substituted Judgement is impossible,

> a surrogate decision maker should use the Best Interests Standard and choose a course that will promote the patient's well-being as it would probably be conceived by a reasonable person in the patient's circumstances.[27]

For the Commission, responsible judges of the child's best interests must assess the following conditions:

(1) The amount of suffering, and the potential for relief

(2) The severity of dysfunction and the potential for restoration of function

(3) The expected duration of life

(4) The potential for personal satisfaction and enjoyment of life

(5) The possibility of developing a capacity for self-determination

These criteria for a Best Interests Standard offer a means of focusing quality of life judgements. When the Commission applies these criteria to judgements about neonatal non-treatment, it divides the issue into three parts, which are related to three types of therapy: clearly beneficial, ambiguous or uncertain, and futile (see Table 2.1).[28]

Table 2.1. Treatment Options for Seriously Ill Newborns
Physician's Assessment In Relation to Parent's Preference

Physician's Assessment of Treatment Options*	Parents Prefer to Provide Treatment**	Parents Prefer to Forego Treatment***
Clearly beneficial	Provide treatment	Provide treatment during review process
Ambiguous or Uncertain	Provide treatment	Forego treatment
Futile	Provide treatment unless provider declines to do so	Forego treatment

As orderly as this classification appears on paper, it obviously leaves one fundamental challenge to those dealing with real cases: how should we decide whether treatment is beneficial, futile or uncertain? This is the question the Commission attempts to answer, or, at least, to guide those who have to make the real decisions for real patients, with all their individuality, complexity and uncertainty.

(1) *Clearly beneficial therapy*: These are treatments for which "there is a medical consensus that they would provide a net benefit to a child".[28] Invoking the Principle of Proportionality, we are asked to subtract the harms of treatment (e.g., the lasting side effects of high-pressure ventilatory support for a premature infant) from the benefits (e.g., extending life). But, more fundamentally, we are instructed to calculate the net benefits of life itself for the permanently handicapped child. The underlying concern of the Commission is that we not produce medical "successes" that are human disasters. Rather, we must honestly consider whether a life-extending treatment is beneficial by courageously asking whether the resultant *life* is beneficial. While urging great caution, the Commission believes the degree of irremediable dysfunction and suffering for some children is so great that life is an intolerable burden, and life-extending treatment would be an unjustifiable injury.

However, for others, and they explicitly focus on the Down's syndrome child with an intestinal blockage, life despite the handicap is a net benefit; and, therefore, withholding life-extending treatment would not be justified.

(2) *Clearly futile therapy*: For some infants, such as the child with a lethal irremediable cardiac anomaly, life is so compromised and so inexorably brief that life-extending heroics could provide no significant benefit, and might well entail significant additional suffering. The patients in this category have lives that "are likely to be measured in hours or days, not years."[29] (The Commission does not explicitly address the non-terminal but permanently unconscious infant.) For such imminently and irreversibly dying patients, life-extending treatment should not be provided. The only exception would be if parents insist on treatment and the child is not suffering.

(3) *Ambiguous cases*: For some patients there is no consensus on whether more life is beneficial or harmful. An example might be a newborn diagnosed with Lesch–Nyham syndrome, who could live a year or so but with progressive disability and suffering. Here the Commission makes three recommendations: (a) Whenever the ambiguity results from factual uncertainty, we must treat until our prognosis is reliable. (b) Ambiguous cases cannot be resolved by "objective" sets of criteria, such as John Lorber's criteria for the non-treatment of myelomeningocele.[30] Such criteria, the Commission insists, conceal subjective value judgements behind an appearance of objective factual determination.

This, however, seems an unfair criticism. Lorber and others who use medical criteria, acknowledge they are making value judgements. Criteria such as birth weight or head circumference or location of spinal lesion are taken as reasonably accurate prognostic markers for future disability. The physicians then consciously judge that certain degrees of disability entail an unacceptable quality of life.[31]

Perhaps the real objection to using a criteria system is not that it conceals subjective judgements but that it strengthens the claim that physicians should be the ones making such judgements. This would reduce the number of cases judged "ambiguous", and thus reduce the number of cases decided by the parents.

This leads us to the Commission's final recommendation: (c) For ambiguous cases, parental judgement should be respected and encouraged. The Commission advocates a *prima facie* acceptance of parental authority and respect for parental autonomy. This is based on our established cultural standards, the practical need for families to be able to handle their lives in their own way in order to be functional, the prevalence of parental benevolence, and their capacity, with suitable assistance, to grasp the significance of medical information and to make realistic and responsible medical decisions. Only when their judgements are clearly and intractably opposed to the care providers' certain judgement of the child's best interests should the parents' judgement be overridden.

One of their strongest recommendations is for the medical partner to put more information into the joint decision-making process. They clearly are concerned that parents at times receive outdated or incomplete information from their physicians, and so are unable to act as informed decision-makers. To deal with this focal concern, the Commission advocates the following steps:

(1) Hospitals should have explicit written policies on decision-making procedures for life-sustaining treatment (Recently adopted as a requirement of the Joint Commission on the Accreditation of Health-related Organizations).

(2) Priority should be given to training caregivers in communication and decision-making skills, with particular emphasis on using an interdisciplinary team to work with the parents.

(3) The institution should establish an Ethics Committee in order to ensure the accuracy of information, the appropriateness of decisions, and the fair mediation of disputes.

The Commission has a basic faith in the reasonableness and goodness of parents and physicians working together. When guided and complemented by community-developed policies and community-reviewed decisions, this surrogate process provides the best possible protection for the best interests of the children whose lives are in our care.[32]

SUMMARY

We began this chapter by asking the question, "When is choosing death for a child justified?" In seeking grounds to stand on when we must take such a stand, we have turned to the positions developed by the major medical, legal and ethical organizations during this last focal decade. Now it is time to ask whether our collegial review has produced, if not hard answers, at least some firm consensus that can help structure and guide our individualized answers to the questions.

I believe that we can indeed discern a useful set of guidelines. However, we should underscore that these do not, for better or worse, go beyond "guidelines". Even the Federal Regulations, which have often been condemned by opponents as moral micro-management, preserve respect for a significant degree of discretionary judgement in custom-tailoring individual decisions. But, there is agreement that we can delineate standards for making meaningful distinctions between better and worse judgements.

To summarize, there are five major components of this well-argued and well-supported consensus:

1. Choosing Death may be Justified

A blind vitalist commitment to doing all for each "life" is generally rejected. So is a fatalistic submission to the terrible genetic errors and traumatic accidents that afflict our children. So is a Technolatrous Imperative, which would let our capacity to *do*, blind us to our responsibility to only do *good*.

Our right, indeed our duty, to make rational and humane choices between extending and ending life is clearly and forcefully affirmed. We owe the real individual children in our care nothing less.

2. Primacy of the Child's Best Interests

To quote once more the synoptic declaration of the American Academy of Pediatrics, "The pediatrician's primary obligation is to the child."[33] The consensus recognizes the reality and intensity of competing interests, including those of the mother and father, siblings, other patients, and other societal needs. However, the inalienable value of the individual child's life prohibits taking that life away for the sake of any other person or cause. Only when life is judged worse than death *for this child*, may we ethically choose death for this child. Only when in good faith we cannot tell which is worse, may we allow the needs of others, particularly those of the child's family as the most immediately and substantively affected, to be weighed on the scales.

3. Ultimacy of the Professional's Judgement

We are taking persons' rights most seriously when we respect their right *to be wrong*: when we support their choices even though we disagree with them. But, the clear consensus is that parents do *not* have such an unqualified right, at least not if their "wrong" choice is to have their child die.

The pediatric professionals' obligation to serve their patients requires them to make their own best judgement of the child's best interests. When this produces a definite judgement for life, parents will not be allowed to overrule the professionals strongly held commitment. Whether explicitly or not, the caregivers' duty to protect a child against medical neglect, including especially fatal neglect, overrides respect for parental choice.

We should note a major omission from all the discussion. None of our guides address the question of whether professionals should be authorized to overrule the parents demand to *continue* life-extending treatment that the physicians judge futile or harmful. Neither, as of this writing, has any court authorized discontinuing treatment and ending a child's life against parental wishes, even in the case of an anencephalic child[34] or a brain dead-child.[35]

4. Medical Conditions Set Limits

It has been said that there are two kinds of people: those who divide everything into two kinds, and those who don't. When it comes to decisions to forego life-support, there are clearly two kinds of people: liberators and regulators.

Liberators believe in the intrinsic sensitivity and responsibility of the involved and invested caregivers, both professional and parental. They advocate individual discretion behind a screen of privacy. They adamantly oppose the impositions of general standards or uniform regulations. They would categorically expel all regulators and other strangers from the bedside.

Regulators, on the other hand, fear the human capacity for ignorant, emotional or self-serving misjudgements of the needs and interests of other persons. Privacy, they fear, may conceal abuse of extremely vulnerable, defenseless children, abuse which is no less deadly because well-intentioned.

For liberators, the most grievous danger comes from the moral tyranny of inflexible absolutes and insensitive procedures. For regulators, the most dreadful harm results from the moral anarchy of uncontrolled judgements with irreversible consequences.

The communal consensus is that the extremes can be avoided by establishing certain medical conditions as the necessary conditions for foregoing treatment. As with any risk assessment, these conditions are chosen because of two factors: severity and probability. The more severely burdened or damaged the child's condition, and the more certain we are of the nature, degree and irreversibility of the child's condition, the more justified we are in letting the child die. The clear intent is to set some degree of objective limit on the notoriously elastic nature of subjective judgements about when a life is not worth living.

The medical conditions that have come to be a clear matter of consensus are:

(a) Terminally ill

(b) Permanently unconscious

(c) Medically futile
(d) Disproportionate burdens of treatment over benefits.

As we have discussed these in detail throughout the chapter, we shall only reiterate our previous claim. Inescapably these are quality of life judgements. While medical conditions may offer some degree of objective check on subjective judgement, we finally must accept the responsiblity of choosing the conditions that we believe are so dehumanized or dehumanizing as to justify terminating life-extending treatment. We must neither ignore nor abdicate from our responsibility for choosing how we make such judgements.

5. Do Not Go Gentle Into That Good Night

There is a clear consensus that we must bear the burden of a demanding process of careful checks and balances in order to responsibly discipline our life-or-death judgements. As appealing as the nostalgic sepia-toned image of a private doctor-patient-family decision may be, this is clearly no longer viable, nor (almost as clearly) permissible. Too many persons are aware and involved in the modern hospital to make privacy possible. And too many factors and views are relevant to make such isolation sufficient.

Two forms of communal checks-and-balances have become commonly required. The first is the use of some form of bioethics committee review. As this is fully explored in Chapter 4, we need only note here that the use of a collegial committee is another attempt to find that balance between the extremes of excessive restriction and excessive discretion.

The second check is to apply an informed consent model to such decisions. This formal structure slows the process down, reinforces the need for conclusively determined and completely documented medical conditions, and reinforces the need for full and thorough discussion of all these demanding elements in order to build the responsive and responsible partnership necessary for such fateful decisions.

CONCLUSION

Those deciding whether to forego life-extending treatment must always search for a very delicate balance between undertreatment and overtreatment, between possibly denying significant benefit and possibly imposing senseless harm.

Since decisions to withhold or withdraw treatment will most likely have fatal, irreversible consequences, our medical and legal and ethical communities have traditionally chosen to err on the side of prolonging medical treatment, and, consequently, human lives. This caution should be even greater when deciding for infants and children. Unlike an adult, most children do not have the capacity to clearly express their own authentic choices. Neither is there a record of previous expressions of their individual values and goals to guide our speaking for them as they would speak for themselves.

To further compound our life-extending inclinations, with children we are tragically denied the usual consolations that strengthen our resolve to make fatal choices for adults. We cannot comfort ourselves with analgesic platitudes about it being “natural”, or “in the order of things". The death of a child is just too unnatural, too out of all sensible, humane order. Neither can we be consoled with a sense that a child's death is timely, occuring only after having lived a "good, long life", and having achieved all that life offers. The death of a child shatters the promise of life, and mocks our puny attempts to find moral order in our mortal sentence.

These are the shadows that make it so dreadfully difficult to see clearly enough when death is right, or, at least, less tragic than a devastated life. In these fateful situations, we do well to turn to those who have borne these burdens and faced these mysteries in order to help guide our own awful choices.

References

1. Roy, D. J. (ed.) (1978). Medical Wisdom and Ethics in the Treatment of Severely Defective Newborns and Young Children. Montreal: Eden Press, p. 37.
2. Koop, C. E. (1977). The Slide to Auschwitz, *Human Life Rev.* **3** (Spring), p. 103.
3. Editorial, New York Times, April 27, 1982.
4. Rudolph, A. M. (1982). Pediatrics, (17th Edition). Norwalk: Appleton-Century-Crofts.
5. Reprinted in 49 Fed. Reg. 1622, 1623 (1984).
6. The Rehabilitation Act of 1973, Public Law 93-112 29 U.S.C. 794 (1982 and Supp. III 1985).
7. Public Law 98-457, 98 Stat. 1749, 42 U.S.C. 5101-05 (1985).
8. Department of Health and Human Services, Final Rule, 50 Reg. 14, 878 (1985) 45 C.F.R. Part 1340.
9. The Child Abuse Prevention and Treatment Act Amendment of 1984 (op cit.).
10. Joyner, N. (1973). Symposium: Child Abuse, *Pediatrics*, 51:799, and Schmitter, B. D., Keimpe, C. H. The Pediatrician's Role in Child Abuse and Neglect. In Gluck, L. (ed.) *Current Problems in Pediatrics*, Chicago, Year Book 1975.
11. Public Law 98-2157 (op cit.).
12. Freidson, E. (1970). *The Profession of Medicine: A Study of the Sociology of Applied Knowledge*, NY: Dodd, Mead & Co. and Moore, W. E. (1970) *The Professions: Roles and Rules*, NY: Russell Sage Foundation.
13. Weil, W. B. *et al.* Committee on Bioethics, American Academy of Pediatrics (1983). Treatment of Critically Ill Newborns. *Pediatrics*, **72**(4):565–566.
14. Committee on Bioethics, American Academy of Pediatrics (1994). Guidelines on Forgoing Life-Sustaining Medical Treatment. *Pediatrics*, **93**(3):532–536.
15. op cit., 565
16. ibid.
17. American Medical Association (1981). Current Opinions of the Judicial Council. Chicago: AMA, p. 8.
18. American Medical Association (1992). Code of Medical Ethics: Annotated Current Opinion. Chicago: AMA, p. 13.
20. Caplan, A., Cohen C. (1987). Imperiled Newborns. *Hastings Center Report*, **17**(6):5–32.
21. ibid., p. 13.
22. ibid., 15–16.
23. McCormick, R. (1974). To Save or Let Die: The Dilemma of Modern Medicine. *JAMA*, **229**(2):172–76.
24. ibid., p. 15.
25. President's Commission for the Study of Ethical Problems in Medicine and Biomedical and Behavioral Research (1982). *Making Health Care Decisions*. Washington D.C.
26. President's Commission for the Study of Ethical Problems in Medicine and Biomedical and Behavioral Research (1983). *Deciding to Forego Life-extending Treatment.* Washington, D.C.

27. ibid., p. 136.
28. ibid., p. 217.
29. ibid., p. 219.
30. Lorber, J. (1973). Early Results of Selective Treatment of Spina Bifida Cystica. *British Medical Journal*, **201**.
31. Lorber, J. (1971). Results of Treatment of Myelomeningocele. *Dev. Med. and Child Neurol.*, **279**.
32. *Deciding to Forego*, op cit., p. 218.
33. Weil, W. B. *et al.* Committee on Bioethics, American Academy of Pediatrics (1983). Treatment of Critically Ill Newborns. *Pediatrics*, **72**(4):565–566.
34. New York Times, February 19, 1994.
35. New York Times, February 18, 1994.

3 Deciding to Let Go: Foregoing Life-Sustaining Treatment for Infants

Alan R. Fleischman

The New York Academy of Medicine, 1216 5th Avenue, New York 10029 and Albert Einstein College of Medicine New York, USA

The decision to forego life-sustaining treatment is a heart-wrenching choice, no matter the age of the patient, the involvement of the family or the experience of the physician. Health care professionals and families alike feel the awesome responsibility when asked to choose whether someone will live or die. It is easy to invoke principles upon which such choices should be made and to describe processes which ought to enhance the outcome but it is hard to actually live through these choices for ourselves, our loved ones, or our patients.

In this chapter, I will use fictionalized cases based on years of clinical experience to illustrate the complexity of bringing principles to practice. I hope to illustrate how the principles of ethical decision-making can help clarify our obligations, support family involvement in the choices and, most importantly, advocate for the interests of the children who are our patients.

Jeff Lyon in his book "*Playing God in the Nursery*" graphically portrays the dilemma that parents and physicians alike encounter — "if it is hard to justify creating blind paraplegics to obtain a number of healthy survivors, it is equally hard to explain to the ghosts of the potentially healthy that they had to die in order to avoid creating blind paraplegics."[1] This tragic trade-off is at the heart of many of the awesome choices we have to make all too frequently.

Monica Madison, a 26-year-old neurosurgical intensive care nurse, was having a "perfect pregnancy" until at 25 weeks gestation (15 weeks early) a sudden gush of fluid, which wet her slacks, indicated rupture of the protective membranes surrounding her fetus. She paged her husband, Dr. Jason Madison, a 29-year-old resident in urology, and they went immediately to consult her obstetrician. Monica was examined, assessed and admitted to the antepartum unit with a plan for conservative management and the hope that the amniotic fluid would reaccumulate, that infection would not occur, and that labor would not commence. During the ensuing two days, Monica alternatively prayed, cried, and talked with her friends and relatives as she complied with the regimen of strict bed rest and continual monitoring and assessment of the fetus. Jason, on the other hand, attacked the problem by gathering all of the information he could from friends and books. He read voraciously concerning the problem of premature rupture of the membranes and the prognosis of 25 week gestation babies.

Unfortunately, after 48 hours, although there were no signs of infection, labor commenced and could not be stopped with tocolytic agents. The obstetrician alerted the neonatal team that delivery of this extremely immature fetus was inevitable. He shared his view with the Madisons that babies of this gestational age rarely survived and generally were left with devastating neurologic sequela. When the attending neonatalogist, Dr. Robert Kaufman, came to the labor floor to visit the Madisons, several hours prior to the birth of the baby, Jason Madison was prepared. He told Dr. Kaufman with his wife concurring through teary eyes, that they wanted no resuscitation of their baby. He had read a great deal about the likelihood of survival and the future quality of life of babies who do survive, and concluded that it was not warranted to impose the severe pain and suffering of technological intervention on this marginally viable child or the overwhelming devastation on the parents.

In a sensitive and caring but very firm manner, Dr. Kaufman informed the Madisons that in this hospital and, he believed in most around the country, fetuses at twenty-five weeks gestation would be resuscitated if live-born and parents did not have the authority to preclude that intervention. He invoked concerns for the child, the hope that this child would not only survive, but would survive with good outcome, and described many such infants whom he himself had treated and followed in the developmental assessment program affiliated with the neonatal unit.

The focus of Dr. Kaufman was on the possibility of a good outcome and his obligation to support that potential. The focus of the Madisons was on the likelihood and consequences of a bad outcome and their fear of how that scenario would impact on them and their soon-to-be-born baby.

As the labor pains continued and intensified, Monica lost control and cried out in anger that she didn't deserve this punishment, that God was being unfair and that her life was about to be ruined. Jason's response, while holding his wife's hand and listening to her outbursts, was an intensification of his anger at being out of control of the circumstances and at being unable to comfort his wife or himself.

Joey Madison was born by vaginal delivery at 10:30 a.m. on Friday morning. He was 680 grams (1 pound 8 ounces) and appeared to be a typical, active, $25\frac{1}{2}$ week gestation, premature infant. The neonatal team in the delivery room intubated the baby to assist with breathing, assigned the initial Apgar score as six at one minute and seven at five minutes, and transferred Joey to the neonatal intensive care unit for stabilization and treatment.

Several minutes later, after Monica had been transferred to the recovery room and was sleeping comfortably as a result of some sedation administered by her obstetrician, Jason arrived in the neonatal intensive care unit to confront the reality of the birth of his son and to discuss the treatment plan with the neonatal team. He continued to request, and even demand, that the doctors stop the aggressive technological intervention. He spoke in clear and rational terms, not losing control nor behaving unprofessionally. The nurses and doctors at the bedside tried to reassure him that Joey was active and vigorous and responding well to the therapy while allowing the distraught father to voice his views and doubts.

However, by the time Monica was able to visit, things were not going as smoothly. Respirator settings had to be increased so that blood oxygen levels would be maintained and the activity which Joey had shown initially was no longer evident. He lay quietly in his open warmer and responded not at all as his mother stroked him while she cried at his bedside.

After rounds on Saturday morning, Dr. Kaufman found the Madisons in Monica's room, distraught, upset and angry. He attempted to describe the positive aspects of the last 24 hours of Joey's treatment and continued to describe the children he had cared for who looked just like Joey did on the first day of life and who were doing well in infancy and childhood. Dr. Madison followed Dr. Kaufman from the room and confronted him in the hallway, arguing that he really didn't care about the other children. He was concerned that his child would be devastatingly impaired and that what was happening now was inappropriate and causing little Joey as well as himself and his wife to suffer inordinately. In an attempt to calm Jason, Dr. Kaufman reassured him that babies of this gestational age frequently declared themselves in the first three days of life, and regardless of what treatments were provided, often succumbed. He assured Jason, as he had assured Monica, that he would keep in close contact with them and he would see them again on Sunday morning after rounds.

On Saturday evening at 6:15 p.m., Dr. Kaufman received a call at home from the neonatal fellow at Joey's bedside. Joey was acutely deteriorating, blood gases were poor, blood pressure was dropping and it appeared clinically that he had developed a major pneumothorax (air leak) on the right side of the chest. The fellow would not ordinarily have called his attending physician to ask what to do; routine procedure would have been the immediate drainage of the air through needle aspiration and the insertion of a plastic chest-tube. By calling the attending at home, the neonatal fellow was figuratively and literally requesting permission to not intervene and to allow little Joey to die from this complication of prematurity and respirator treatment. In addition, the fellow and the attending physician alike knew that the occurrence of a pneumothorax in the early stages of the care of the small premature infant is highly correlated with significant intraventricular hemorrhage-bleeding in the brain. A pneumothorax with cardiovascular deterioration in a premature infant who, heretofore, was unresponsive, significantly increases the likelihood of the ultimate death of the child or a very poor future quality of survival. Nevertheless, Dr. Kaufman insisted that a chest tube be immediately placed and, in fact, returned to the hospital to assure that Joey would receive excellent resuscitative efforts to both reverse the respiratory problems and to re-establish normal blood oxygenation and blood pressure.

On Sunday morning, even before Dr. Kaufman could enter the neonatal intensive care unit for rounds, Jason Madison was waiting to talk with him. Dr. Madison argued that not only was the treatment prolonging an inevitable dying process and causing extraordinary suffering for Joey, but that the entire therapy was experimental. He argued that none of the treatments had been proven effective for infants of this gestational age and weight, and therefore, he as the father ought to have the right to refuse all clinical experimentation. Dr. Kaufman listened calmly and reassured Jason that Joey was responding well to the treatments and although the therapies were not always successful, they were a standard part of neonatal care in units such as this one.

Early Monday morning a portable ultrasound examination of Joey's brain revealed severe intraventricular and parenchymal hemorrhage. These findings were completely consistent with the clinical course and physical findings in this small premature infant. Although not certain, hemorrhage of this extent in this type of patient is associated with a very high likelihood of death or exceedingly poor quality of future life. Dr. Kaufman noted on rounds with the staff that morning that although this was a very bad sign, there were patients he had seen with similar bleeds who did very well with mild to moderate retardation and cerebral palsy. When asked by the nurse whether the ultrasound findings would make Dr. Kaufman reconsider the Madisons' request for stopping of treatment, he brusquely replied that he would not abandon Joey just because his parents didn't want him.

Four days later, after another pneumothorax and an unsuccessful attempt at aggressive resuscitation, Joey did die. Monica and Jason Madison received the information at home and cried with deep sadness at the loss of their son and relief at the end of their ordeal.

This complex, but not atypical, case raises several important issues which will need to be explored. Prior to delivery, is there a role for advance directives? Are do-not-resuscitate orders for infants who are about to be born necessary in order for physicians to refrain from aggressive intervention? Are these orders sufficient to obligate physicians not to resuscitate an infant who appears to be viable and would likely benefit? After delivery, what is the appropriate role of parents in making treatment choices for their newborn? What responsibility does the physician have to advocate for his view of the interests of the baby and how much weight should be given to the parental request for discontinuing treatment? What level of certainty of ultimate outcome is required before a physician may advocate for letting a child die, or allow parental choice in that regard? Does the possibility of a good outcome, however slim, obligate physicians to advocate for continued treatment? Is neonatal intensive care experimental when it is applied to marginally viable infants?

Before I address these questions, this case must be contrasted with another which illustrates how differently concerns and values may be balanced by decision-makers for newborns.

Sally Brown was admitted emergently to the hospital labor and delivery suite in active labor at what was thought to be 24 weeks gestation. Sally was 18 years old and although a senior in high school, had been unable to continue her education because of this pregnancy. She had received three prenatal visits at a community clinic where no problems had been reported. Although Sally had a history of smoking and drinking with her friends on the weekends, she had taken her responsibility to her future baby seriously and had not engaged in these practices after she learned she was pregnant. Labor progressed rapidly and there was no time for the neonatal team to speak with or even to meet Ms. Brown. Her son was born at 2:00 a.m. on Wednesday. He weighed 580 grams (1 pound $4\frac{1}{2}$ ounces) and appeared to be approximately $24\frac{1}{2}$ weeks gestation. Apgar scores were two at one minute and five at five minutes. He was intubated, resuscitated and transferred rapidly to the neonatal intensive care unit for stabilization. Four hours later, at about 6:00 a.m., the neonatal fellow and pediatric resident who had been present throughout the little boy's life, reported to his mother that he was stable. They informed her that he was on a respirator, had received medication to enhance his breathing, that there was some chance that he could survive and that if he did make it there was some chance that he could do well. Sally listened but heard very little. She continued to ask, "Will my baby live?" and "When can I see him?" The doctors repeatedly answered the first question with the hope that he would survive, not quite appreciating that the question encompassed far more, including "Is that good or bad?" Sally waited for her boyfriend, George Roman, to arrive at the hospital before she could muster the strength to come to the neonatal intensive care unit. Mr. Roman, a very young-looking 21-year-old man, was employed as a bicycle courier to hand-deliver critically important business mail. George and Sally visited the baby just after the nursing change of shift at 7:30 in the morning. Linda, the day-shift primary nurse, explained all of the equipment and attempted to reassure the parents that everything was being done for their son. Sally was frightened and overwhelmed by the size of the baby, his appearance, and the intimidating nature of the intensive care environment. George remained cool and aloof, but proud to be the father of a little boy. They named the child George, Jr., GJ for short, and began immediately to call him by name.

Sally and George desperately wanted GJ to do well. They visited frequently and heard only the positive comments from the doctors and nurses caring for the baby at the bedside. GJ moved, responded to touch and the suctioning of his mouth and airway, and required no medication to maintain his blood pressure. However, by the third day of life, two ominous events had occurred. Brain ultrasound revealed a severe grade IV bleed in the ventricles, extending to the substance of the brain. In addition, chest X-ray showed worsening lung findings with what appeared to be a very early, but severe, sign of chronic disease.

As Dr. Martha Ramirez, the attending neonatologist, arrived at her office just outside the neonatal intensive care unit on the morning of GJ's fourth day of life, she was greeted by the head nurse of the night shift. She had stayed behind an extra half hour awaiting Dr. Ramirez's arrival in order to be certain that the attending physician heard her perceptions about the appropriateness of withdrawing treatment from GJ. The head nurse reported that Sally and George had visited from about 9:00 p.m. to about 2:00 a.m. that night and had wept openly at the bedside, lamenting the fact of GJ's worsening breathing problems and his devastating brain damage. The head nurse informed Dr. Ramirez that the family was clearly prepared to withdraw treatment and allow GJ to die and would arrive sometime this morning to discuss their decision with the staff in the unit.

Dr. Ramirez reviewed all of the facts of GJ's medical course on rounds at the bedside. She discussed the present treatment plan and shared her ambivalence and uncertainty with the doctors and nurses. She agreed that the likelihood of GJ's surviving was very slim, and if he did, the likelihood of extremely poor outcome with prolonged hospitalization and severe disabilities was virtually certain. As a physician, she was reluctant to withdraw the present treatments, hoping instead to have the opportunity to withhold a future needed intervention which would result in the death of the child. She was prepared, however, to sit with the family, discuss their feelings, and to generate a plan which might ultimately result in the death of GJ.

George and Sally arrived around noon bringing with them Sally's stepfather, Fred Johnson. The three family members were ushered into a small conference room in the neonatal intensive care unit where Dr. Ramirez, the neonatal fellow, the pediatric resident, the neonatal social worker and the primary nurse for GJ, were quickly summoned. A discussion ensued in which Dr. Ramirez explained the very serious nature of the impact of the profound prematurity on GJ and the very small likelihood of survival. Mr. Johnson spoke first, saying that they were a very religious family who believed that God would heal GJ and that there were forces far greater than the doctors and nurses that would determine the outcome of his grandson. When asked, Sally and George echoed Mr. Johnson's views, and insisted that they wanted "everything" to be done to enhance the likelihood of GJ's survival.

The social worker, Mr. Longwood, and Dr. Ramirez were quite surprised at what had transpired during the meeting. Dr. Ramirez had prepared herself to agree to withdraw treatment and allow GJ to die, yet the family was now requesting everything be done, a complete turn of events. Mr. Longwood requested that Sally stay behind so that he and Dr. Ramirez could speak to her privately while Mr. Johnson and George visited with GJ in the unit. Sally reaffirmed in private the views she had voiced at the meeting. She wanted GJ to live and she wanted the doctors and nurses to do everything possible to make that happen. She cried and revealed that she understood that he might survive with significant impairment, but she believed that God would help her son and that he would ultimately thrive and lead a normal life. Dr. Ramirez and the other staff in the neonatal intensive care unit reassured Sally that they respected the right of parents to make these choices and they would comply with her wish to continue aggressive interventions in an attempt to save GJ's life.

Although Mr. Johnson never returned to the neonatal unit, Sally and George visited regularly. GJ went through virtually all of the serious complications of prematurity: heart failure, inflammation of the bowel, multiple and repeated infections, and hydrocephalus (a swelling of the internal fluid-filled areas of the brain). Once or twice each week Dr. Ramirez or the senior neonatal fellow would sit with Sally, or Sally and George, and explain the current problems and the treatments. Several times Sally had been called and told to come to the hospital because GJ was deteriorating rapidly and it looked like he might die. Each time with increasingly aggressive measures, he responded and stabilized. He never improved, but he continued to persist. With each of the deteriorations and at each of the weekly meetings the neonatal staff again raised the question as to whether new treatments should be withheld or present treatments withdrawn. Each time Sally responded by requesting that "everything" be done to support her son. Reluctantly, but diligently, the professionals in the neonatal unit continued to provide aggressive treatment to GJ.

At the end of GJ's second month of life, Dr. Ramirez rotated off the service and Dr. Michael Gold became the attending neonatologist of record. His first impression upon reviewing GJ's case, discussing the course of treatment with the staff and examining the patient, was that further treatment of GJ was clearly futile. In his opinion, GJ could not survive and if he did survive, which was very unlikely, he would be severely impaired and virtually vegetative. Therefore, he believed that continued treatment was inappropriate and should not be provided. The social worker, the nurses in the unit, as well as the other physicians explained to Dr. Gold that although Dr. Ramirez had been willing to withhold or withdraw treatment from GJ on many occasions dating all the way back to the first week of life, that the family had insisted on treatment and that their request had been respected. Dr. Gold replied non-verbally and basically became passive in the care of GJ. He rounded daily and examined the patient, but rarely commented on the plans generated by the pediatric residents and neonatal fellow. He spoke politely to Sally and George when they visited, but he did not continue the weekly meetings that had occurred with Dr. Ramirez.

GJ died that month, not for lack of life-extending care, but because all of the doctors and nurses had been correct in their belief that even with aggressive treatment GJ would inevitably die. The final event was his fourth episode of sepsis, with generalized cardiovascular deterioration unresponsive to various medical interventions. At the very end, Sally allowed GJ to be taken off the respirator so that she could hold him as he died in her arms. She reported to the nurses that she felt satisfied they had done everything they could, and that she had done everything she could for her son.

Dr. Gold on rounds the day after GJ's death talked about another case he had been involved with some years previously. In that case, a child close to brain dead, vegetative from the first day of life, had been kept alive for six months at the request of the family. He had been appalled that resources had been utilized in this way and had believed that physicians had an obligation to not squander dollars that could be used far more productively for the health care needs of other children. Dr. Gold went on to explain that GJ's care had cost well over $150,000. Had he been allowed to die on the fourth day of life, enough money would have been saved to pay for the multi-channel apnea monitoring system the unit so desperately needed and had been requesting for well over a year from the administration. He implied that he would not have been as gracious as Dr. Ramirez in allowing the parents to determine the extent of the treatment provided, but he gave no explanation as to how he would have behaved differently, and which treatments he would not have provided.

This second case adds several important questions. Is there an ethical distinction between withholding and withdrawing treatment? What counts as an acceptable rationale for determining what is in the interest of the child? When does further treatment become futile? May physicians or parents make a unilateral decision as to whether treatment should be continued?

These cases bring stark reality to the theoretical framework for health care decision-making for infants and children. It is easy to articulate the principle of "best interest" and to explain the obligations that physicians and parents bring to making choices for children, but it is hard to define what is the right choice and the right process in individual cases. However, careful analysis of these vignettes may allow for some conclusions that can be generalized or are at least helpful in assisting professionals and parents alike in decision-making for critically ill children.

Because critically ill infants are unable to articulate or advocate for their own interests, it is important that there be societal safeguards to assure that these vulnerable patients are protected.[2] Parents are given a wide latitude in our society to decide what enhances their child's well-being in areas ranging from housing, clothing, nutrition, and religion, to health care decision-making. This is based on the belief that parents are the appropriate decision makers for their children and that they have an identity of interests with their child.[3]

Health care professionals also have an important role to play in assessing what is in the interest of their patients. When patients cannot make autonomous choices and have not previously voiced their preferences, which is the case for all infants, physicians have a greater obligation to assess what is in the interest of the patient and to advocate for these interests when critical choices must be made. Health care professionals have an independent obligation to their infant-patients to advocate for their well-being by assuring that the decisions are based on the patient's best interests.[4] These obligations require judgements, independent of family wishes, concerning what is the right choice for the child. Physicians stand as societal representatives to assure that the choices parents make for the health of their children are within a range of acceptable options and based on a reasonable assessment of the interests of the child.

I firmly believe that virtually all parents love their children and wish their children to be healthy and happy members of our society. As such, parents can and do assess what they believe to be in the best interest of their child. In the complex cases in which there is conflict concerning the right choice for a critically ill child, parents quickly realize that what is in the best interest of their child is often unclear and uncertain. When parents and health care professionals disagree, it is most often the case that there exists no single objective criterion to guide their judgment.[5] It is not appropriate to attempt to resolve this dispute by creating the fiction of asking what a child who has never had decision-making capacity would choose if lucid or capable for the moment. This approach may be helpful for formerly capacitated adults who may have voiced their preferences when capable, or expressed their values in how they lived. This is called making a substituted judgement, that is, we make the choice we believe the patient would likely make, regardless of our personal view of the right choice.[6] For infants, however, an individualized choice must be made which places the infant's interests as central, neither denying the child legitimate treatments, nor forcing the child to endure inappropriate interventions. How we accomplish this goal is the crux of this chapter.

While parents are the appropriate decision-makers for their children, we must not expect parents who love their child to be so separate and aloof as to be able to objectively define the interests of that child without at the same time having their own interests affected. Parents must take into account their own feelings, the impact of this decision on their lives and on other loved individuals in the family. The complexity of making these best-interest judgments by an individual parent for a critically ill child requires us to explore the thoughts and feelings of the parent and to understand better the multiplicity of concerns which enter into the final decision.

We should not allow parental desire to avoid emotional, financial, or other hardships to deny clearly beneficial medical care to a critically ill child. However, we should not trivialize the importance of these issues to the family nor should we ignore the need to provide social supports to mitigate these concerns. Parents are most often aware of these internal conflicts and are willing to enter into the struggle to avoid sacrificing the interest of their critically ill child to the interest of themselves or their other loved ones. We can help parents to be aware of these potential and real conflicts through sensitive and thoughtful communication and openness to these ambivalent feelings. This exploration generally results in a decision firmly grounded in the interest of the patient. However, disagreement about the right choice may occur between parents and professionals. In most instances in which conflict arises the disagreement between parents and health care professionals concerns whether continued survival in a debilitated or burdened condition warrants continued treatment. This should be acknowledged as an honest value-conflict.

Health care professionals also have great difficulty in making an objective assessment of the interest of their patient. Physicians also bring personal values and experiences to their decisions. Professionals respond to their awesome responsibility in varying ways. Some wish to maintain control of the decision-making, some are worried that they will be criticized for their decision, others are concerned that the death of a patient is a failure, and others are burdened by a desire not to inflict undue pain and suffering on their patients. Each of these feelings may be present when health care professionals play an important role in health care decision-making for children. It is important for each health care professional to explore his or her own values and motivations when attempting to define the best interest of an individual patient. Health care professionals rarely consider their own feelings and have difficulty admitting that they are uncertain as to what is in the interest of their patient. However, physicians should be able to explore their own feelings, assess their motivation, and come to a decision which places the interest of the child as primary. Because of the training and experience of physicians, as well as their professional distance from their patients, we have the right to expect that they will be more objective in their views about the right choice for the child. This should place them in a position to help counsel parents and to assist the process of making the decision which best reflects the child's interest.

Physicians, as was the case in our two vignettes, are generally quick to judge parents who disagree with their perceptions of what is in the best interest of the child, whether it be requests for non-treatment or requests for all treatments for a critically ill child. Although we may disagree with a parent's perception of what is the right choice for their child, we must maintain our respect for their views and values, even when we do not agree and cannot concur. Respect of an opinion does not imply capitulation. We should remember that reasonable people may disagree concerning the right choice when there are real value conflicts.

With this grounding in the clinical reality and human complexity, I will address some of the questions raised by the cases. In the first case, the parents did not wish their unborn child to be resuscitated at the time of delivery. Some have argued that this request should be respected based on the analogy to the family's right to request a do-not-resuscitate order for their loved ones who do not have the capacity to decide for themselves. However, in virtually all situations in which a physician agrees to a surrogate's request for a do-not-resuscitate order, that physician has assessed the patient's medical condition and concurs that non-resuscitation is a reasonable choice. Surrogate decisions for incapacitated patients which will result in the death of the patient, unlike autonomous choices of capacitated patients, are usually limited by the medical condition of the patient as assessed by the physician.

Because of the uncertainty of the circumstances of an individual delivery, and the need to assess the patient before making the decision as to whether or not to resuscitate, I believe that a do-not-resuscitate order prior to delivery is inappropriate and unnecessary. It is inappropriate because the health care professional has an independent obligation to the patient which requires that an assessment be preformed on the newborn infant in order to decide whether resuscitation is appropriate. Do-not-resuscitate orders prior to delivery are also unnecessary because clinicians have no obligation to resuscitate those infants for whom treatment would not be beneficial. In addition, if resuscitative efforts are initiated, parents ought to be reassured that treatment can be withdrawn if the infant is not responding or is not benefiting from the intervention.

Most health care professionals continue to believe that withholding a treatment which results in the death of a patient is more appropriate and certainly easier psychologically than withdrawing a treatment. There is no question that there is a psychological difference between not starting and stopping. But, when the motivation of the decision is the ultimate death of the patient, it is harder to find an ethical or legal distinction. In addition, it has been argued recently that initiating treatment with the intent of stopping if the therapeutic trial proves non-beneficial, is more appropriate than withholding a therapeutic intervention entirely.[7] In the first vignette, I believe that resuscitation in the delivery room and initial stabilization of the infant in the neonatal intensive care unit was appropriate treatment. However, as the infant deteriorated and the benefits of continued treatment became marginal and uncertain, parental choice ought to have been respected. The attending physician initially appeared motivated by a well-meaning desire to preserve the possibility of a good outcome. In my opinion, he insisted on continued treatment because he believed that allowing a child to die who might have been normal is a far greater evil than continued treatment for a child who might survive in a devastatingly impaired condition. It is, however, unlikely to be reassuring to parents that a physician has seen a good outcome in a similar case when the most probable and likely outcome is poor. It is highly likely that parents will view this optimistic assessment in a different manner as was the case in the vignettes described.

The reasons that parents bring to their choices and the values which they hold, may not be viewed as fully rational by the intellectual calculus of the physician. Belief in spiritualism and forces greater than science and medicine or the acceptance of severe disability as a part of humankind, are values held by many of our patients and their families. These values were respected in the second case and resulted in the continued treatment of the child even though ultimate death or severe disability was likely. We have socialized physicians to accept parental choice when continued treatment is the desired outcome, even when the health care professional disagrees with the decision. Since the primary justification for medical intervention on a child is the ability to benefit the patient, not the parents, health care professionals sometimes feel constrained by the ethics of their profession to resist requests for continued interventions that may provide only marginal benefits to their patient. If a requested treatment cannot benefit a patient, it should be considered futile, and the health care professional has no obligation to provide it. If, however, the benefit of the treatment is possible, although unlikely, this creates a more complex dilemma.

Physicians often use the term "futile" or "not beneficial" when a treatment is unlikely to cure or enhance the future quality of a patient's life. This use of the term futile is inappropriate.[8] I believe a treatment is futile if it cannot benefit a patient in the narrow, strictly physiologic sense. If a treatment can support the prolongation of a patient's life for more than a few hours or days, it may be of questionable benefit and even not in the patient's interests, but should not be called futile. The language of futility is often used by physicians in an attempt to arrogate to themselves the choice of whether to provide a treatment. Physicians may not wish to provide such a treatment based on their perception of what is in the best interest of their patient and may even wish to opt out of the care of such a patient by transferring such care to another physician; but, they ought not to attempt to preclude the parental role in the choice by calling a marginally beneficial treatment "futile."

I have found that the hardest cases to resolve even with consultation, are those in which the family is requesting an intervention which is at best only marginally beneficial to the child, and at the same time, increases the pain and suffering of the patient. These are, thankfully, very rare cases; but, in such circumstances physicians understandably will object to inflicting pain for a low likelihood of benefit. Those who strongly object should be encouraged to transfer the care of the patient to another professional more willing to accept that level of marginal benefit for the burden imposed. In some rare cases, bioethics consultation or even court intervention, may be appropriate to protect the child. In general, however, the marginal potential benefit of continued treatment ought to be respected while the physician makes certain that the patient does not suffer by using the appropriate medication to alleviate pain and anxiety.

While physicians have attempted to arrogate choice to themselves through futility language, parents may also attempt to arrogate to themselves the sole right to make the choice by invoking the concept of "experimentation". Some have argued that neonatal intensive care and other risky interventions with a low likelihood of a successful outcome are clinical experiments rather than therapy. Participation in clinical research has always been viewed as optional and requiring the full and informed consent of the patient or in the case of children, of the parent or legal guardian. Clinical interventions which are experimental require assessment by independent review committees and may be refused without question by families. Because the goal of research is to ascertain whether a clinical intervention is effective, this basic uncertainty as to outcome requires that there be no obligation on the part of the patient or family to consent to the research. Although many interventions in the neonatal intensive care unit are of high risk and some are of low likelihood of success, most have been subjected to experimental verification and ought not to be considered clinical research. This does not mean that parents ought not to have the right to decide whether they wish their child to be the subject of such interventions, but the choice ought not to be based on the assertion that these therapeutic interventions are, in fact, experiments.

I have attempted to argue that the arrogation to the physician, or to the parent, of the sole right to choose the treatment for an individual child are both inappropriate. How then ought we to resolve these complex conflicts between well-meaning parents and well-intentioned physicians? It seems apparent that merely invoking the best-interest principle or the language of beneficent obligations will not help resolve these real value-conflicts. It is possible, however, to move closer to resolution of these dilemmas by encouraging open communication among the participants in the decision, and by the acceptance of all parties of the inherent value conflicts which are at the basis of the disagreements. Physicians ought not to view their duty as blind advocacy for any chance of the continued life for their patients. Parents ought to be given wide latitude in their choices, particularly when the likelihood of benefit is marginal or uncertain. When conflict arises, consultation by an ethicist or ethics committee as well as the assistance of other knowledgeable professionals in the clergy and mental health fields may be helpful in resolving these disputes.[9]

The basic goal is collaborative decision-making.[10] We must place the child, as much as possible, in the center of the analysis in an attempt to ascertain his or her interests. At the same time, we must accept a wide variation in views and values related to this assessment. Exploring the values which are in conflict and causing disagreement between families and professionals and among the different professionals can be helpful in the ultimate resolution of the dilemma. The goal should not be making identical decisions in all medically similar cases. Rather, acceptance of differing family values will result in different decisions in medically similar cases out of respect for parental views, beliefs and wishes. This approach is consistent with our respect for personal values and family autonomy while still protecting the rights and interests of the child.

When physicians wish to discontinue treatment over the objection of the family, they often invoke the squandering of societal resources as the rationale. This was part of the lament of the physician at the end of Case 2. Although resource allocation questions are important, particularly in this era of health care reform and cost-consciousness, invoking these economic concerns at the bedside is inappropriate. The societal decision as to what level of neurologic capability warrants expenditure of resources, ought to be a choice made at the conference table or the ballot box and not at the bedside. In addition, I believe that if society is going to decide that some patients are so gravely ill or disabled as to not warrant the expenditure of societal resources, these choices should be made for patients of all ages, not just infants. Society, through its democratic processes, could decide that when a patient, regardless of age, sex, race, or economic standing, is determined to be in a specific medical condition, such as a persistent vegetative state, then further treatment will not be provided. Such a decision would not be in the hands of either the individual family or the physician, but would be societally determined and uniformly applied.

Some physicians and other commentators believe that the money saved by not treating a critically ill child will go directly to preventive interventions or provide needed equipment for intensive care units. This view is incredibly naive in the present financial structure of the health care system. There is no reason to believe that money saved by the withholding or withdrawing of treatment from a newborn in a neonatal intensive care unit will result in the immunization of a poor child in the community or the purchase of a needed piece of equipment for that unit. It is certainly appropriate for physicians and others who are making choices concerning technologic interventions for patients not to squander precious resources and to be aware of the colossal amounts of money which are being spent on such treatments. However, we should not sacrifice the lives or interests of individual patients to the misguided belief that individual physicians can reallocate the dollars from these expensive technological interventions to needed preventive services.

Ultimately, the most appropriate decisions for our children who are gravely ill will be made through a process of communication and values exploration between the health care professionals responsible for the care rendered to the patient and the parents of that child. The community pediatrician, family practitioner, or other health care professional with a relationship to the family and an interest in the care of the child may be extremely helpful in counselling the family, mediating disputes, and advocating for the interest of the child. In the first vignette, the attending neonatologist showed disdain for the parents' desire to stop treatment and argued that he would not let the patient die just because his parents didn't want him. The community pediatrician with a relationship to these parents might well have been able to impact on the attending neonatologist's view by both giving social support to the parents and explaining to the neonatologist that they were behaving in a manner which deserved his respect and consideration, even if he could not agree with their conclusion. In the second case, in which the parents were insisting that everything be done in support of their child and eventually voiced relief at having provided ultimate parental support by doing everything that they could for their child, the community pediatrician could have been supportive of the parents' views, while helping them to reassess the balancing of the potential benefits of continued treatment with the possible burdens inflicted on the child. An additional reassuring presence by the practicing pediatrician in the lives of the young parents might have allowed them to accept that they had done "everything" for their child and still might have allowed treatment to have been stopped far earlier.

I believe it is important for the community pediatrician and other health care professionals who are part of the lives of critically ill children to be involved in the decision-making process to forego life-sustaining treatments. Given the nature of modern neonatal intensive care, these professionals may not be the direct caregiver; but, because of their position of respect from both the health care professionals and the families, they may serve as important mediators and consultants in these difficult decisions.

What else can we do to facilitate an optimal process of decision-making which enhances the interests of critically ill and vulnerable neonates? There should be regular discussions in neonatal units of the ethical issues inherent in health care decision-making for infants. One method to accomplish this goal is through ethics rounds on a weekly or monthly basis.[11] These teaching conferences allow for the training of all professionals in the exploration of the potential value conflicts which may arise in the neonatal unit. In addition to these and similar educational opportunities, open communication between the professionals and parents can be fostered by frequent and regular meetings to share views on progress and prognosis. Time should be allocated to allow parental reaction, response, and questions. In cases where ethical conflicts seem likely, consultation should be sought early in the process, before the development of adversarial relations.[9] Whatever systems are developed or adapted to facilitate dialogue, the most important part of the process is the ability of physicians to be sensitive to their own values and to respect the views and values of others who also care about their patient.

Society places responsibility for the well-being of vulnerable children in the hands of their parents. Health care professionals are asked to shepherd this relationship and assist in its nurture. Children can be thankful that they are profoundly cherished by their families and that to a major extent they are valued by our society. Children should not be fearful that they will be devalued and allowed to die inappropriately because their parents or their physicians are not concerned with their best interest. Additionally children should not be fearful that they will be used to fulfill the desires of others and inappropriately forced to live burdened lives of inordinate suffering. Decisions to forego life-sustaining treatment can and should be made for children through a process which places their interests as primary and respects their parents' views and values. Health care professionals should continue to be the ultimate arbiters of these choices, thoughtfully fulfilling their obligations to the children without unduly imposing their own values on patients or families.

References

1. Lyon, J. (1985). *Playing God in the Nursery.* New York: W. W. Norton.
2. National Commission for the Protection of Human Subjects (1979). *The Belmont Report*, Washington, D.C.: U.S. Government Printing Office.

3. Duff, R. S. and Campbell, A. G. M. (1973). Moral and ethical dilemmas in the special care nursery. *New England Journal of Medicine*, **289**:890–894.
4. Gaylin, W. and Macklin, R., (Eds) (1982). *Who speaks for the child: The problem of proxy consent.* New York: Plenum.
5. Rhoden, N. K. (1986). Treating Baby Doe: The ethics of uncertainty. *Hastings Center Report*, **16**:34–42.
6. Buchanan, A. and Brock, D. W. (1986). Deciding for others: Standards for decision making. *Millbank Quarterly*, **64:Supp12**:67–80.
7. Hastings Center (1987). Guidelines on the termination of life-sustaining treatment and the care of the dying. New York.
8. Truog, R. D., Brett, A. S. and Frader, J. (1992). The problem of futility. *New England Journal of Medicine*, **326**:1560–1564.
9. Fleischman, A. R. (1987). Bioethical review committees in perinatology. *Clinics in Perinatology*, **14**:379–393.
10. Fleischman, A. R., Nolan, K., Dubler, N. N., *et al.* (1994). Caring for gravely ill children. *Pediatrics*, **94**:433–439.
11. Fleischman, A. R., Arras, J. (1987). Teaching medical ethics in perinatology. *Clinics in Perinatology*, **14**:395–402.

4 Pediatric Ethics Committees

Sanford Leikin[1] and Jonathan D. Moreno[2]

[1]*Children's Hospital, National Medical Center, 111 Michigan Avenue N. W., Washington D.C. 20010-2970, USA*
[2]*SUNY Health Science Center at Brooklyn, 450 Clarkson Avenue (Box 116), Brooklyn, New York 11203, USA*

INTRODUCTION

Ethics committees are a novel way to pursue moral problems in health care facilities. These committees have arisen from societal and professional concerns about clinical outcomes, often in connection with the use of newer medical technologies concentrating on pediatric facilities. This chapter will describe how these committees began and how they have developed, their constitution and operation, and it will provide guidelines for their evaluation.

ORIGIN AND GROWTH OF PEDIATRIC ETHICS COMMITTEES

Before the 1970's, groups of physicians and other professionals conferred on specific ethical issues, particularly sterilization, abortion, and allocation of scarce medical resources. In 1974, Institutional Review Boards (IRBs) were established by the National Research Act (Public Law 93-348) to examine the scientific and ethical aspects of human subjects research. During the 1970's a few hospitals formed committees to review cases in which the withholding or withdrawing of life-sustaining treatment was being considered.

The public's attention was first attracted to the concept of hospital ethics committees through the case of Karen Quinlan, a 21-year-old comatose woman whose parents sought legal sanction to have her respirator removed. The court ruled that, before it could be removed, an "ethics committee" should agree that "there is no reasonable possibility of Karen's ever emerging from her present comatose condition to a cognitive, sapient state."[1] In its ruling, the court referred to an article written by a pediatrician, Dr. Karen Teel, an advocate of ethics committees. Dr. Teel described an advisory, interdisciplinary group to help physicians make "ethical judgements which we are sometimes ill-equipped to make."[2] She suggested that these groups, "composed of physicians, social workers, attorneys, and theologians," provide advice by meeting in a "regular forum" for dialogue on difficult cases. However, the Quinlan court actually proposed a committee composed entirely of medical specialists to give a prognosis about Karen's neurologic status. It is not clear that the court was aware of this substantive difference.

A milestone in the promotion of ethics committees in hospitals caring for either children or adults was the 1983 recommendation of the President's Commission for the Study of Ethical Problems in Medicine and Biomedical and Behavioral Research.[3] Its report stated that having an ethics committee in a hospital "would ensure that an individual or group whose function is to promote good decision-making review the most difficult cases." A pediatric ethics committee could serve several useful functions: confirm that the best information available is being used; assure the propriety of a decision made by parents and physicians; and settle disputes among decision makers. Furthermore, using these committees to promote good decision-making within an institution might prevent exposing these sensitive situations to the adversarial process of the courts.

Another important event promoting the formation of pediatric ethics committees was the issuance of the "Baby Doe" regulations.[4] The regulations followed professional and public controversy about the selective non-treatment and death of a baby with Down's syndrome. These rules made "the withholding of medically indicated treatment from a disabled infant with a life-threatening condition" an instance of medical neglect. While the original Baby Doe regulations which prohibited discrimination against "handicapped" infants were invalidated by the Supreme Court, the Congress subsequently passed an amendment to the Child Abuse Law (P.L. 98-457) which contains much of the intent and language of the original Baby Doe rule. To implement this law, the Department of Health & Human Services (DHHS) published final regulations which encourage, but do not mandate, the establishment of hospital-based committees, called Infant Care Review Committees (ICRC), to assure that disabled infants receive "appropriate" medical treatment.[5]

As a response to the proposed rule, the American Academy of Pediatrics (AAP) advanced the concept of forming bioethics committees in hospitals caring for disabled infants. Composed of pediatric professionals and others, these committees could "provide education, develop and recommend institutional policies, and offer consultation to providers and families facing a range of ethical problems or questions about medical treatment of infants."[6]

The AAP guidelines urged that committees assume a multidisciplinary approach. Expertise available to the committee through members or advisors should include medical, psychosocial, human service resources, nursing, social work, and familiarity with legal and ethical issues affecting disabled persons. The suggested "core" committee members are: a pediatrician knowledgeable about the nursery; a nurse; a hospital administrator; a parent of a disabled child; a representative of a disabled group or a developmental disability expert; a social worker; a member of the clergy; a lawyer; a lay community member; and a person trained in ethics or philosophy. The recommended committee functions were: educating hospital staff, infants' families, and the community; recommending to the hospital's governing board policies for the care of critically ill infants; and retrospective case reviews.

The AAP guidelines also suggested that prospective consultative case review be done "in a voluntary context". The scope of the committee's discretionary review should include the following: the care of a hospitalized infant upon the request of any member of the hospital staff or member of the infant's immediate family when a serious ethical issue is presented by a decision about the infant's care; and review of any case of a hospitalized infant when serious ethical questions about the infant's care have been raised by a public agency.

Within pediatric institutions, some individuals also began to recognize a need for ethics consultation in complex and controversial decision-making.[7] This recognition was sparked by a wish to prevent adverse publicity about the hospital, to avoid political disputes among staff members, or to avoid getting involved in costly and contentious litigation. Additionally, some strongly believed that ethics committees would improve the caliber of decision-making about ethics and diminish the risk that decisions would retrospectively be perceived as unethical.

These events have led to a rapid growth in ethics committees which deliberate about ethical problems arising from the medical care of infants, children, and adolescents in hospitals and other health care institutions. The proposed panels have been given a variety of names: Pediatric Ethics Committee, Institutional Ethics Forum, Institutional Ethics Committee, Ethics Advisory Group, Pediatric Review Committee, NICU (neonatal intensive care unit) Committee, Bioethical Ethics Committee, Infant Bioethics Committee, and Infant Care Review Committee (ICRC). In a 1985 poll by the American Academy of Pediatrics, 66% of the hospitals had infant care committees, up from 56% in 1984. [8]During 1992 the National Association of Children's Hospitals and Related Institutions (NACHRI) surveyed 80 pediatric freestanding and non-freestanding institutions. Some 78% had a pediatric ethics committee. Of the 18 respondents who stated that they did not have an ethics committee, most indicated that pediatric ethics issues were handled by the general hospital ethics committee or an executive committee with pediatric representatives.[9] Another survey noted a correlation between hospitals having a neonatal intensive care unit (NICU) or a pediatric intensive care unit (PICU) and having an ethics committee.[10] A commitment to teaching has also been found to be an important attribute related to establishing an ICRC.[11]

COMPARING PEDIATRIC AND ADULT COMMITTEES

There are medical, legal, and ethical differences between the contexts of adult and pediatric committees. Although the medical differences are most pronounced in neonatal ethics, the maturing human being at any stage presents different challenges for medical management than adults. Legally, the minor child is not presumed to have the authority to make treatment decisions, unless he or she falls into an exceptional group in that particular jurisdiction, such as an "emancipated" or "mature" minor. Further, minors generally do not bear legal responsibility for financial obligations that have been incurred in the course of their treatment. Lacking financial leverage, they perhaps do not have as much of an opportunity to insist upon the satisfaction of their treatment preferences.

Of far greater complexity is the moral status of children in terms of their capacity to make or participate in medical decisions that directly affect them. This is the uniquely challenging area for pediatric ethics committees. Unlike adults who can now, or did in the past, express their personal choices, children and early adolescents have never developed the cognitive and emotional skills needed to formulate and express a set of personal values or preferences. Absent decisional capacity, ethical standards have been formulated for surrogates to decide for them. These are discussed below. In some cases, however, children are able to participate to some degree in medical decisions, and the pediatric ethics committee will need to assess how best to weigh that degree of ability as an expression of respect for the child or adolescent patient.

In our society we do not regard parents as the "owners" of their children, but rather as their trustees until they reach adulthood.[12] Only if parents are abusive or neglectful do they lose some of their prerogatives. Under those circumstances, just as all of society serves as a steward for children, the pediatric ethics committee can be viewed as an agent of this stewardship. In spite of the many similarities between adult and pediatric committees, the unique moral responsibility of pediatric ethics committees seems especially poignant.

ORGANIZATION AND OPERATION

Authorization and Membership

Authorization by the hospital leadership gives ethics committees the formal legitimacy that they require. A survey of 58 pediatric hospitals revealed that 55% were medical staff committees, 38% were established by the administration, 7% by the board of directors, and 1.8% were free standing.[11]

The legal status of ethics committees is evolving. In general, as an agent of the health care institution the ethics committee can be held responsible for the soundness of its procedures, theoretically including the actions of its individual members. In theory, too, the records of ethics committee proceedings are discoverable in a court of law. Thus, care should be taken to ensure not only that the committee conducts itself in a thoroughly professional manner, but also that members are duly appointed and that they are covered by the institution's insurance. This will not normally be a problem for those members who are full-time employees of the hospital, but coverage should be extended to other members drawn from the community.

Appointments to the committee are made by the group that authorized it, usually in consultation with the committee chairman. To some extent, committee membership will depend on whether it deals only with neonates, with all pediatric age groups, or with patients with chronic disabilities. Since the medical and moral questions associated with each of these populations differ somewhat, the expertise required will vary. However, most committees are multidisciplinary. They consist of physicians, nurses, social workers, clergy, bioethicists, hospital administrators, psychologists, school teachers, and community representatives who are often the parents of handicapped or previously hospitalized children.[11,13] The diversity of views provided by these individuals with different expertise and social backgrounds adds significantly to the richness of the committee deliberations. But, as

Cross and Churchill note, "[Although] diversity within the committee is important in defining the broad context, it will be the maturity and wisdom of the individuals that will lead to better opinions, not their diversity *per se*."[14]

Both pediatric generalists and specialists (including surgeons) can be valuable members of these committees. Since most committees review cases involving neonates, the presence of a neonatologist is usually necessary. A disability or physical medicine specialist is also a valuable addition, particularly if the committee is associated with a chronic care facility.

Many committees also include lawyers in their membership. Others have resisted this move, arguing that the presence of a lawyer might focus the discussion on the legal aspects of the case, thus precluding ethical deliberation. Or, as suggested by Kliegman *et al.*, legal counsel might produce a conflict of interest between institutional interests and the ethical role of the committee.[15] The latter reservation has also been expressed about hospital administrators.[16] As members, their institutional bias may unduly influence a committee's deliberation to the detriment of patient or family interests. On the other hand, their cooperation and support is necessary for the committee's effectiveness. When these reservations are serious, these professionals are not made regular members, but are invited to attend only for a specific reason.[15]

Members drawn from the community can be of special value to a bioethics committee. They can contribute to it in various ways. Community members are likely to express a greater degree of subjectivity than the professionals on the committee. As members of a particular culture, they can express a sense of the values and needs of that group. As consumers, they can inform the committee of the concerns of those who must negotiate with health care professionals to receive their services. As parents, they can indicate their thoughts and feelings as advocates for the child, and represent how other parents might think when faced with a particular ethical dilemma. As parents devoted to the care of a disabled child, they can inform committee members about their own and their child's particular needs and burdens, and those of others in similar situations. All of these representations by various kinds of community members contribute immensely to the humanistic character of a pediatric bioethics committee.

Committee Functions

The major functions of pediatric bioethics committees are threefold: (1) case consultation and review, (2) education, and (3) policy development.[6,13,17] These three roles are interconnected and vary in degree among committees, but their essential goal is to facilitate or optimize ethical decisions about infants, children, and adolescents.[15] They are described further in the following sections. Owing to the complexity and sensitivity of case consultation and review, our presentation of this subject will constitute the bulk of the remainder of this chapter.

1. Case consultation and review

Ethics case review is the best-known function of most pediatric ethics committees. Review is most often prospective, although retrospective review is also done by some committees, particularly for teaching purposes.[6,15,18] Three fundamental principles of contemporary bioethics guide committee deliberations.[6,14] They are beneficence, the obligation to benefit, or at least not to do harm; autonomy, the obligation to respect the choices of others; and justice. The first principle prevails when the patient is a neonate or young child. Here, the child's best interest is the primary moral concern. For example, in a child with overwhelming pneumocystis pneumonia secondary to HIV infection, would it be in the child's best interest to continue with aggressive treatment if the child's long-term prognosis seems bleak? Parental autonomy is considered next, because parents generally have their child's best interest as their own priority, and they (next to the infant) are most touched by the decision. But, at times, as in cases of the children of Jehovah's Witness parents, their autonomy may be overridden for the sake of their children. The principle of autonomy can also apply to older children and adolescents: honoring their decisions shows respect for their developing competency. Justice becomes significant to the extent that decisions made for the patient may impinge on the welfare of others.

In pediatric patients of all ages, the most common question brought to ethics committees is whether to forgo life-sustaining treatment, (e.g., surgery, a respirator, dialysis, nutrition and hydration). The reviews have involved premature and full-term infants, and young children with a variety of congenital conditions, (e.g., chromosomal abnormalities, congenital heart disease, myelomeningocele, metabolic disorders), and acquired states, (e.g., birth asphyxia, brain hemorrhage, hepatic failure, HIV infection, necrotizing enterocolitis, and bronchopulmonary dysplasia).[13,15,19] In older children and adolescents, case reviews usually involve patients with acquired conditions, (e.g., malignancies, HIV infection, and brain damage due to trauma) or end-stage disease (e.g., cystic fibrosis).[14,15]

The frequency of prospective case reviews varies among committees. One group reports a total of 31 patients for whom consultation was requested from August 1984 through December 1988, with an average of eight per year since June 1985.[19] In another report, a complex of four university-affiliated hospitals conducted 30 patient consultations in the first 30 months of its existence.[18] A third report describes 11 case reviews in a period of 15 months.[15] At the Children's National Medical Center in Washington, D.C., the committee reviewed 40 cases between its inception in 1984 and 1993. Various aspects of the case review function will be elaborated in the following sub-sections: (a) The review process; (b) achieving a consensus; (c) making a recommendation; (d) assessing ethics committee case review; (e) other ethics consultation models; and (f) staff attitudes toward ethics consultation.

(a) *The review process*

The way in which committees initiate and conduct case review is extremely important for appropriate ethical decision-making and acceptance of the committee within the institution. The elements entailed in the process are: (1) how the committee is accessed for case review, i.e., whether review is mandatory or optional; (2) who may request a case review; (3) who may participate in the review; (4) how the case review process operates; and (5) whether the committee determination is advisory or mandatory.

The guidelines for infant bioethics committees drafted by the American Academy of Pediatrics state that the "committee should review all cases in which the attending physician and parents propose to forego life-sustaining treatment for an infant." Instead, most committees have chosen to make review optional.[13,17] This arrangement has been chosen because many physicians and parents might resent being compelled to have a consultation, thereby discouraging use of the committee mechanism. Furthermore, it is unlikely that consultation would be enforceable in most hospitals. Most important, however, is that most committees view themselves as advisory bodies to which the principals voluntarily come to seek guidance rather than a directive.

Review is usually initiated by contacting the chairman or other committee member. In most institutions, case reviews can be requested by any member of the health care team directly involved in the patient's care, by the family, or by the patient. They are usually asked to resolve ambiguity or disagreement regarding ethical aspects of treatment decisions, or to provide support by sharing decision-making responsibility.

Attendees at case reviews usually include ethics committee members and the medical, nursing and social work staff members involved in the patient's care. Any other medical or surgical specialists who can inform the group about the patient's present or possible future state should also be invited.

It is strongly recommended that the patient, if appropriate and feasible, and the patient's parents be notified about the case review and that they be encouraged to be involved in the deliberation. The parents' contribution to the committee's discussion is extremely important. They can relate their understanding of the child's medical and emotional state, and their expectations about his or her outcome. They can inform the committee about their choice concerning treatment and the reasons for making it. With the parents present, it is also sometimes possible to clarify misunderstandings or ambiguities. Most salient, however, is that it enables the parents to be heard, thereby recognizing and respecting their role as advocates for their child. Indeed, parents will rightly be suspicious of any committee processes that do not make them collaborators in decision-making. In addition to the parents, persons who can help support them, e.g., other family members and clergy, should also be encouraged to attend.

When parents attend case review, care must be taken to limit the number of professionals (and committee members) in attendance. The presence of a large number of strangers reduces the gathering's privacy, and may intimidate parents or make them suspicious that the review is not intended for collaborative decision-making. Under these circumstances, parents are less likely to share their thoughts and feelings, thus diminishing the opportunity for open discussion. Some committees ask the patient's caregivers and the parents to remain for the entire meeting while others excuse them at some point.

During a case review several important objectives should be met: (1) all the relevant medical and psychosocial information is gathered; (2) everyone, particularly the patient (when capable) and family members, have an opportunity to express their views; (3) a careful and thoughtful ethical analysis is made; (4) a consensus is developed; (5) and a recommendation is given.

In the case review, the relevant medical information should include the nature of the child's illness and prognosis, when known. The level of the child's awareness and degree of suffering should also be determined. Alternative treatments should be discussed, including their probable outcomes, their expected risk of harms and any potential benefit.

It is also important to learn as much as possible about family members and their circumstances, their perception of the child's illness and its outcome, and their preferences (or, if the child is an adolescent, his or her wishes). Any misconceptions that the parents may have about the child's illness or its outcome should be ascertained. Further support and counseling that the parents might need, whether their child lives or dies, should also be identified.

Kliegman *et al.*[15] provide a comprehensive list of principles that are useful for guiding the ethical judgements in reviews:

1. Competent patient preferences are to be respected.
2. If the patient is not competent, his or her best interests are the primary moral consideration.
3. When the best interests of an incompetent patient remain impossible for health care professionals to clarify, the family's interpretation of those interests should be respected.
4. The family's own interests and preferences should be considered, but second to those of the patient.
5. Substantial doubt of outcome for the patient favors continuing support.
6. Confidentiality is to be respected so long as it does not jeopardize the best interests of the patient.
7. Committee recommendations are based on moral rather than legal, economic, or political considerations.

These principles recognize that in making such decisions, parents are mindful of the child's best interests and have significant knowledge of non-medical factors bearing on those interests. In fact, both moral and legal traditions of the United States give parents presumptive authority over the welfare of their children. If there is a question, those who would replace parents with another decision-maker must bear the burden of proof for why this should be done.

Besides applying a set of principles, the ethical analysis requires a standard for decision-making. At least two different standards have been suggested: the "best interests" of the patient and the patient's "relational potential".[20] According to the best-interests standard, decision-makers are obligated to determine whether to use or to forgo life-sustaining treatment by weighing the benefits and harms of the treatment and its alternatives. The child's parents and health care professionals are both expected to play a role in making the decision. In determining the child's best interests, care must be taken not to employ a standard that is based on the perspective of unimpaired adults who might not want to live a life with mental or physical disabilities. In order to be as objective as possible, a child-centered quality of life standard should consider whether, from the child's point of view, continuing this life with its impairments would be on balance beneficial or harmful for the child. Unfortunately, we do not have the luxury of comparing his life to a normal existence; for such a child, it is a question of life with impairments, or no life.

However, some children may be so severely neurologically damaged (e.g., coma or persistent vegetative state) that they lack any potential for human relationships. Such children might be regarded as having no interests at all, except perhaps to be free from pain and discomfort. In this case the best-interests standard is not applicable: continued treatment would neither benefit nor harm the child. Instead, the relational potential standard becomes the relevant criterion. This standard is non-obligatory; it allows the withholding or withdrawing of life-sustaining treatment from children who lack the potential for human relationships, but it does not require that treatment be foregone. Unlike the best-interests standard, which is child-centered, the relational potential standard allows the interest of others, e.g., family or society, to weigh in the decision of whether to treat.

(b) *Achieving a consensus*

The literature on ethics committees strongly indicates the preference among committees for consensus as the outcome of their deliberations. Owing perhaps to the inherently philosophical nature of many of the problems they consider, most committees appear to regard voting as inappropriate in the vast majority of situations. Indeed, the impression should not be given that ethical issues can be "decided" in some straightforward manner by democratic means. Furthermore, like other committees, ethics committees are likely to have more influence in the institution if they do not appear divided. Finally, collegial working relations within the committee could be jeopardized by demands that each member take an explicit position on difficult moral questions. If the committee cannot achieve what it regards as a relatively defined consensus, it may wish to identify a range of acceptable alternatives, or suggest some alternative decision-making procedure to the health care team and the parents.

(c) *Making a recommendation*

As suggested earlier, the role of most pediatric ethics committees is advisory, not executive. Thus, it is appropriate that the result of their deliberations be a recommendation to the concerned parties rather than an order. A consensus can lead to several different kinds of recommendations, depending on the circumstances of the case. In some cases a recommendation is given to withhold or withdraw treatment, or whether the treatment (e.g., surgery or blood transfusion) that is proposed or being provided is appropriate.[13,15,21] In other instances, the recommendation involves who should make a decision.[22]

Rather than make a specific recommendation about treatment or about who is to decide, the group may describe what practices fall into an ethically acceptable range, and perhaps state what it believes to be the preferable course of action. At times, because of ethical ambiguity, a committee may not be able to arrive at a consensus concerning the child's best interest, and thus is unable to make a specific recommendation. As suggested, when the latter occurs the family's decision should be honored.[15]

Whenever it appears that the recommendation to be given will be morally unacceptable to a health care provider, it may also be appropriate to suggest that the patient be transferred to another caregiver who is willing to follow the recommendation.

Since ethics committees are not primary decision makers, their recommendations are not binding on either of the involved parties.[17] Nonetheless, after a recommendation is made, it should be presented to the child's parents and the responsible caregiver(s). It is preferable to do this by meeting separately with each party, and not only stating the recommendation but also providing the committee's reasons for it and answering any questions that may arise.

If disagreement remains after the recommendation is given, the appropriate hospital authority is apprised of the matter. At this point the ethics committee has fulfilled its advisory function. Following review of the issue, if the hospital authorities agree with the committee's recommendation, they may direct caregivers to follow the recommendation. Caregivers are free to withdraw from the case, so long as an appropriate transfer of care is possible. If parents disagree with the recommendation, the hospital authority can pursue legal action in order to obtain a court order. If the hospital authority remains undecided about which view to support, a judge may be requested to rule on the matter.

Minutes of the case review are kept by most committees. Additional documentation varies among committees. Some record the recommendation or a summary of the proceedings in the patient's chart, while others only state that a consultation was done, or leave the decision of whether to enter a note in the chart up to an administrator or the attending physician.[18,19] Recording a summary of the case review or the recommendation in the patient's chart has the advantage of enlightening interested staff members who are unable to attend the review.

(d) *Assessing ethics committee case review*

Ethics case review offers several potential benefits. It provides the opportunity to subject moral dilemmas to group discussion, thereby incorporating the input of a variety of persons and reducing the influence of any one perspective. It also can enhance communication between the involved parties. Furthermore, the process can assist in ethical decision-making by ascertaining relevant facts that may clear up misunderstandings which sometimes develop among physicians, nurses, social workers, and family members. It may also give reassurance to staff members and parents that a good decision is being made. Other possible advantages that the committee affords are: (1) helping the participants appreciate and respect the views and values of others; (2) suggesting strategies to prevent or reduce conflict with parents; (3) establishing a range of ethically acceptable options; and (4) alerting staff members to those decisions that are clearly unethical or illegal.

Despite these possible advantages, a careful assessment of the value of ethics committee case review in pediatric decision making has not been conducted. One possible way to accomplish this task would be to compare this decision-making context with the established method of decision-making employed in judicial review. However, the adversarial nature of judicial proceedings differs from the strategy employed in ethics case review. A more appropriate comparison might be clinical decision-making practiced in everyday encounters between physicians and their patients or their families. This would require a systematic description of how decisions are made in the absence of committees. Moreover, the problem with making this kind of comparison is that the cases reviewed by ethics committee are not like those found in everyday encounters. They are usually of a higher order of complexity and are laden with emotion.

At this time, instead of trying to make either of these comparisons, it is more important that we develop a better understanding of the case review process and outcome.[23,24] For example, who knows about the committee's existence and its accessibility for case review? What are the avenues of access to the case review? Are they available to all staff members, patients, and families? What are the social, ethical, and legal reasons for seeking case review? Why are certain cases presented and others not? Which of the involved parties is invited, and who attends the case review and who does not? What is the review process like, and how are committee recommendations formulated?

The actual effect of case reviews also needs to be reviewed. When committees make recommendations about patient care, are they followed? When they are followed, is it because of convincing reasons presented by the committee, or because of the perception of the committee's authority, or fear of legal liability? Lastly, but of extreme importance, research is needed to determine "user satisfaction." Are members of the hospital staff, patients, and parents satisfied or dissatisfied with the case review process and why? In what ways do they think the review process could be improved?

(e) *Other ethics consultation models*

Besides the formal bioethics committee case review described above, other methods of providing consultation are available in some pediatric institutions. These modalities can be provided independent of, or in conjunction with a committee. Grodin and associates describe a three-member team which functions independently of a committee.[25] It consists of a physician with formal training in ethics and health law, a hospital attorney with a background in social work, and a hospital administrator with a public health and patient advocacy orientation. In addition to providing consultation at the request of hospital staff, patients or parents, the team has extended its role to policy formulation and to the establishment of educational programs.

Michaels and Oliver describe the use of rotating on-call teams consisting of a physician and a non-physician who are members of a committee.[26] These teams provide consultation on an optional and advisory basis. Recommendations made by the team are subsequently reviewed by the entire Human Rights Committee.

In addition to the team approach, consultation can be provided by single individuals. A number of hospitals caring for adults use this method.[27] This modality has not been reported as being used to any great extent in pediatric institutions. Nevertheless, the ethics committee at one of our institutions has established a consultation service and continues to explore its use. When the chairman of the ethics committee has been contacted about an ethical issue concerning a patient, an assessment is made of its urgency and degree of complexity. If the issue can be readily resolved by the chairman giving reassurance, providing information about hospital policy, or encouraging that a patient care conference be held to improve communication among staff members, a formal case review by the committee is not convened. If such consultations do not require the committee at that time, they are still reviewed retrospectively at its next regular meeting.

(f) *Staff attitudes toward ethics consultation*

Currently, little is known about how hospital staff members view ethics consultation by a committee or a team. A survey of 238 community-based and full-time attending physicians at the Children's Hospital of Pittsburgh found that 29% had requested a consultation.[26] It also indicated that hospital-based physicians and those who admit more patients are more likely to request a review. In 48 consultations, the reason most often stated for the request was to "facilitate" decision making, but other important reasons were to clarify moral issues and to help provide legal protection. The principal reasons physicians gave for not seeking consultation were that they had not encountered an ethical dilemma or that they did not know about the existence of the service.

Another survey of physicians and nurses who attended prospective case reviews suggests that the majority of these professionals considered them helpful.[23] They thought that the meetings resulted in a clearer awareness of ethical principles relevant to the cases discussed, and that they increased the likelihood of better decisions. The survey indicates a favorable perception of ethics committees, but Mahowald does not believe that it demonstrates that case reviews do, in fact, improve the quality of ethical decisions. She states,

> Quality may be defined in terms of consistency with applicable ethical principles... A study to determine whether infant ethics committees (IECs) improve decisions in this regard would require examination of decisions in similar cases from a representative sample of institutions, comparing those that do and those that do not utilize IECs.[23]

2. Education by the Ethics Committee

Three forms of education are provided by ethics committees. Most important is the committee's self-education. It is conducted in several ways: supporting members' attendance at bioethics meetings, distributing current literature on bioethics, inviting outside speakers, and conducting retrospective case review and analysis.

Education is also directed toward hospital staff to inform them about hospital policy on ethical matters and on ethical principles and analysis so that ethical decision-making can be improved. It can be provided by lectures, conferences, and rounds. Our own experience and that of others indicates that the case-oriented method is best for teaching medical and nursing graduates.[28] In addition, publications about ethical issues, e.g., newsletters and reprints, can be provided to staff members. Besides the hospital staff, families are informed about the means and resources available within the hospital and in the community to assist them in ethical decision making, including the availability of the ethics committee and how to access it.

An additional educational role of pediatric ethics committees is in community outreach. Increasingly, the public is being confronted by difficult ethical dilemmas occurring in the treatment of infants and children. It is important that it be educated about them and their complexities, and encouraged to deliberate on them and develop a consensus about them. Because of their expertise with these ethical issues, pediatrics ethics committees can play a useful function in this dialogue.

3. Policy Recommendations

Many pediatric ethics committees develop and recommend hospital policy and guidelines on ethical matters. This activity is important in establishing a hospital's moral attitude. Such policies may concern a variety of issues. For example, the ethics committee of one author's institution (S.L.L.) has drafted and recommended to the hospital board policies on the following: (1) foregoing life sustaining treatment, (2) DNR ("do not resuscitate") orders, (3) the use of anencephalics for organ donation, and (4) the employment of HIV-positive health care professionals in the institution. The AAP Infant Bioethics Task Force and Consultants recommends writing guidelines for specific kinds of cases or diagnoses, e.g.,

Down's syndrome or myelomeningocele, but not all committees have embraced this proposal.[6,15]

Case review frequently involves considering whether futile treatment is being provided to the patient. This has led some committees to write, or consider writing, a policy concerning the provision of futile treatment. Such a policy might allow the withdrawal of treatment which is deemed futile. As there have been no commonly accepted criteria for characterizing this term, the ethics committee at one author's institution (S.L.L.) has concluded that at present it is not wise to write such a policy. Instead, we intend to educate staff members about the vagueness of the concept of futility, and to encourage and educate them in conducting shared decision making with patients and families.[29]

QUESTIONS AND ANSWERS ABOUT ETHICS COMMITTEE

At first blush, bioethics committees appear to be a valuable resource in pediatric institutions, but many questions and concerns have been raised about them. Some of the following remarks about these issues are derived from the literature on ethics committees in institutions caring for adults. Nonetheless, the similarity in constitution and function between committees in adult and pediatric institutions also makes these comments applicable to pediatric ethics committees. The major concerns are: (1) the awareness of hospital staff members about the committee's existence; (2) accessibility and participation in committee proceedings; (3) subversion of the proper authority of parents or professionals by a committee; (4) the potential for committees to be bureaucratic; (5) the possibility that committee deliberations are biased toward institutional interests; and (6) the possible tendency for them to develop "groupthink".

A problem of accessibility to a committee may result from a lack of awareness by staff members of its existence.[30,31] For example, one recent study of five Maryland general hospitals indicates that a substantial proportion of physicians, house officers, nurses, and social workers did not know of their committee's existence.[30] Of these groups, physicians were least likely to know. As mentioned earlier, a principal reason that staff and community physicians gave for not utilizing the pediatric ethics committee at the Children's Hospital of Pittsburgh was ignorance of its existence.[26] Aside from that single exception, we lack knowledge about the level of awareness of staff members concerning the presence and availability of the services of the pediatric ethics committee in their hospital.

Concern has also been expressed about the extent to which patients and families are allowed to be involved with ethics committee deliberations.[32,33,34] Agich and Youngner suggest that the involvement of patients and families is complicated by ambiguity in the understanding of what ethics committees are all about.[33] These authors identify six different types of access: (1) knowledge of the committee's existence and function; (2) awareness of specific committee meetings or consultations; (3) consent for specific case review to occur; (4) convening the committee or initiating a case review; (5) attendance at ethics committee meetings and direct involvement in ethics consultations; and (6) access to reports and recommendations.

At a minimum, it would seem that all parties with a direct relationship to the child or adolescent patient (and in some cases the patient himself or herself) should be aware that the committee is considering an ethical issue that involves the patient and should have access to the committee. This is a fundamental element of the legal principle of due process and serves the ethical principle of respect for the patient and his or her parents and caregiver. Therefore, efforts should always be made to notify the parents of the case review, and, when appropriate, to encourage their attendance. On the other hand, it is not inconsistent for the committee to insist that some of its deliberations are to be closed if this can be justified as most likely to serve the child's interests.

In general and in the long run, everyone will be best served if openness and candor characterize the committee's involvement. One author has commented that as her pediatric ethics committee has developed, more parents have been invited to be involved in case review.[19] Yet, other than this fragmentary information, we do not know how pediatric ethics committees are conducting themselves in relation to the six types of access mentioned above.

Skepticism about the involvement of a committee in matters traditionally decided by parents and physicians is wholly understandable. As for any consultative individual or group in the hospital, only if the committee is likely to make a contribution to the patient's well-being can its involvement be justified. Since pediatric ethics committees are involved only at the request of some party directly responsible for the child or adolescent patient, if it conducts itself professionally and sensitively, there should be little basis for concern about its role. Furthermore, since any recommendation made by the committee is not binding on the involved parties, their decisional authority is not compromised.

Another problem related to committee case review is their potentially bureaucratic nature. Siegler is concerned that ethics committees will subvert the physician–patient relationship and inflict administrative burdens on patients' families and their physicians; that physicians will yield decision-making power or that the committee will usurp the physician's role; and that decision-making will be distant from the clinical setting, becoming disinterested and bureaucratic, and that a conflict of interest with administrative needs will arise.[35] To what degree pediatric ethics committees intrude into the role of physicians and families in decision-making has not been determined. Nor do we know whether the decisions that committees make are less compassionate than those at the bedside. However, including the patient's care team and the parents in the ethical deliberation, and striving to apply the qualities of an "ideal observer" — knowledgeable, thorough, disinterested, dispassionate, and consistent — offers the best opportunity to diminish their bureaucratic tendency.[7]

Concerns about bias toward institutional interests must be addressed in several ways. First, there must be a general understanding by the administration that, although defensive legal practices may seem beneficial in the short run, in the long run all will be best served if the patient's interests are taken as paramount. Second, whatever the administration's role in the membership and proceedings of the committee, its influence must be carefully monitored. Third, committee members who are not employees of the institution have an important role as guardians of this understanding. Finally, the committee's integrity will ultimately be judged by the manner in which it meets its responsibilities to those who are being cared for by the institution and its staff.

The concern that, like any small group, an ethics committee's deliberations are subject to distortion or "group think", has been raised in the literature.[34] Perhaps the greatest threat is that a few influential members will succeed in dominating discussions and imposing their view on others, e.g., those with the highest professional and social prestige, (usually male physicians). Here the skill of the chairperson as a facilitator becomes critical in ensuring that no single point of view is accepted at face value, and that all views are fully heard and carefully weighed.

CONCLUSION

Ethics committees in pediatrics exhibit all of the novelties and uncertainties of health care ethics committees generally. In addition, they are involved with decision-making for children, a population that has exceptional emotional significance, and one that is also uniquely vulnerable. The burden upon pediatric ethics committees is thus considerable. It is far too early to tell with certainty whether they will succeed in their goals. Yet some experience has accumulated that can provide guidance for the future, and that leads us to commend this experience to those engaged in the care of children.

References

1. Supreme Court of New Jersey. *In re* Karen Quinlan, an alleged incompetent, 70 N.J. 10, 355 A2d 647.
2. Teel, K. (1975). The Physician's Dilemma. *Baylor Law Review*, **27**:6–9.
3. President's Commission for the Study of Ethical Problems in Medicine and Behavioral Research (1983). *Deciding to Forgo Life-Sustaining Treatment.* Washington, D.C.: U.S. Government Printing Office pp. 153–255.
4. U.S. Department of Health & Human Services, Office of the Secretary (July 5, 1983). *Nondiscrimination on the Basis of Handicap Relating to Health Care for Handicapped Infants.* Fed. Reg. 48. No. 129.
5. Federal Register 49 [1984, 14873-14892].
6. Infant Bioethics Task Force and Consultants (1984). Guidelines for infant bioethics committees. *Pediatrics*, **74**:306–310.
7. Fost, N. (1992). Infant care review committees in the aftermath of Baby Doe. In: *Compelled Compassion.* Caplan A. L., Blank, R. H., Merrick, J. C., (Eds.) Totawa, NJ: Humana Press.
8. Fost, N. (1986). What can a hospital ethics committee do for you? *Contemporary Pediatrics*, **3**:119–129.
9. We are grateful to Ms Dorothy Albritton of the National Association of Children's Hospitals and Related Institutions for providing this information.
10. Fleming, G. V., Hudd, S. S., LeBailly, S. A., Greenstein, R. M. (1990). Infant care review committees: the response to federal guidelines. *Am. J. Dis. Child*, **144**:778–781.
11. Levine-Ariff, J. (1989). Institutional ethics committees: a survey of children's hospitals. *Issues in Comprehensive Pediatric Nursing*, **12**:447–461.
12. Bartholome, W. G. (1981). The child–patient: do parents have the "right to decide"? In: Spicker, S. F., Healey, J. M., Engelhardt, H. T., (eds.) *The Law–Medicine Relation: A Philosophical Exploration.* Dordrecht, The Netherlands: D. Reidel.
13. Leikin, S. (1987). Children's hospital ethics committees: a first estimate. *Am. J. Dis. Child*, **141**:954–958.

14. Cross, A., Churchill, L. (1986). Pediatric ethics committees: learning from our experience. Editor's column. *J. Pediatr.*, **108**:242–243.
15. Kliegman, R. M., Mahowald, M. B., Youngner, S. J. (1986). In our best interest: experience and workings of an ethics review committee. *J. Pediatr.*, **108**:178–188.
16. Levine, C. (1984). Questions and answers about hospital ethics committees. *Hastings Centre Report*, **14**:9–12.
17. Fost, N., Cranford, R. E. (1985). Hospital ethics committees: administrative aspects. *JAMA*, **253**:2687–2692.
18. Fleischman, A. R. (1987). Bioethical review committees in perinatology. *Clin. Perinatol.*, **14**:379–393.
19. Edens, M. J., Eyler, F. D., Wagner, J. T., Eitzman, D. V. (1990). Neonatal ethics: development of a consultative group. *Pediatrics*, **86**:944–949.
20. Special issue on imperilled newborns: standards of judgement for treatment. *Hastings Centre Report*, Dec. (1987) **17**(6):13–16.
21. Weir, R. F. (1987). Pediatric ethics committees: ethical advisers or legal watchdogs? *Law, Med & Hlth Care*, **15**:379–403.
22. Fleischman, A. R., Murray, T. H. (1983). Ethics committees for Infants Doe? *Hastings Centre Report*, pp. 5–9.
23. Mahowald, M. B. (1992). Baby Doe committees: problems in evaluation. *HEC Forum*, **4**:5–18.
24. Greiner, G., Storch, J. (1992). Hospital Ethics Committees: Problems in Evaluation. *Hospital Ethics Committee Forum*, **4**(1):5–18.
25. Grodin, M. A., Markley, W. S., McDonald, A. E. (1985). Use of an institutional ethics team on a pediatric service. *QRB* pp. 16–19.
26. Michaels, R. H., Oliver, T. K. Jr. (1986). Human rights consultation: a 12-year experience of a pediatric bioethics committee. *Pediatrics*, **78**:566.
27. Fletcher, J., Quist, N., Jonsen, A. (1989). *Ethics Consultation in Health Care*. Ann Arbor MI: Health Administration Press.
28. Pellegrino, E., Hart, R., Henderson, S., Loeb, S., Edwards, G. (1985). Relevance and utility of courses in medical ethics: a survey of physicians' perceptions. *JAMA*, **253**(1):49–53.
29. Benrubi, G. I. (1992). Futility. *South Med. J.*, **85**(3):299–302.
30. Hoffman, D. (1991). Does legislating hospital ethics committees make a difference? A study of hospital ethics committees in Maryland, the District of Columbia, and Virginia. *Law, Med. & Hlth. Care*, **19**(12):105–119.
31. Nash, R., Leinbach, M., Fought, R. (1989). The hospital ethics committee: who knows it exists and how to access it? *HEC Forum*, **1**:9.
32. Mozdierz, G., Reiquam, W., Smith, L. (1989). Shaping access to hospital ethics committees: some critical issues. *HEC Forum* **1**:31–39.
33. Agich, G. J., Youngner, S. J. (1991). For experts only? Access to hospital ethics committees. *Hastings Centre Report*, pp. 17–25.
34. Lo, B. (1987). Behind closed doors: promises and pitfalls of ethics committees. Sounding board. *NEJM*, **317**:46–49.
35. Siegler, M. (1986). Ethics committees: decisions by bureaucracy. *Hastings Centre Report*, pp. 22–24.

5 Tell All the Truth? Shepherds, Liberators, or Educators

Robert C. Cassidy

Schneider Children's Hospital-Long Island Jewish Medical Center, 269-01 76th Avenue, New Hyde Park, New York 11040, USA

Tell all the Truth but tell it slant —
Success in Circuit lies
Too bright for our infirm Delight
The Truth's superb surprise
As Lightning to the Children eased
With explanation kind
The Truth must dazzle gradually
Or every man be blind —

Emily Dickinson

INTRODUCTION

In practice, most Pediatric ethics has been "Trickle-Down Ethics". That means the baseline values and dynamics in medical ethics have been defined by the adult patient-doctor relation. Adult rights based on adult capacities and roles have provided the normative model. Then, to the extent that the minor patient is believed to have become adult-like, he or she is granted adult-like rights and roles. Consequently, while almost all other compenents of Pediatrics have come to appreciate and respect the unique nature and needs of the child, Pediatric ethics is still treating the child as a "little adult".

Truth-telling is the perfect example of this approach. Whether truth is granted to children is determined by an adult's judgment of the degree of their intellectual capacity to understand, emotional capacity to handle, and social capacity to use the truth appropriately. The assessment of the adult-like status of the child determines how much truth will be "awarded".

Since most children do not have either the capacity (or the clout) of the fully endowed adult, and since adults have traditionally been comfortable deciding for children, the dominant role for pediatric caregivers has been that of the "Good Shepherd", committed to protecting their vulnerable, immature charges from the burdens and risks of hard truths and tough decisions.

The Shepherds have been opposed by two other major views about the appropriate allocation of truth and choice to children. The "Liberators" stand on the opposite end of the spectrum. Insisting that each child is a unique individual person, Liberators assert a duty to respect and support the rights of children as fully as those of older individuals.

The third view, that of the "Educators" is a uniquely pediatric model. The Educators fall somewhere in between the very protective Shepherds and the very empowering Liberators. The Educators' model is based on a developmental understanding of children. Recognizing that the essential dynamic of childhood is the development towards maturity through the practice of adult roles and skill, the Educators call pediatric caregivers to promote the child's growth in understanding, coping and choosing by providing age-appropriate opportunities for practicing these challenging tasks.

This chapter will analyze the arguments and logic of the Shepherds, Liberators and Educators' answers to that classic ethical question: "How much should we tell our young patients?"

To focus our understanding of the issues, we shall begin by considering the actual policy and practice of a pediatric oncology service at a children's hospital.[1]

OKLAHOMA CHILDREN'S MEMORIAL HOSPITAL ONCOLOGY SERVICE

(1) ***Initial Conference***: All children four and older will be included, with parental consent. Parents will be urged to consent.

Children will be told they have cancer.

They will be told the nature and side-effects of the therapy.

They will be told that without therapy they will die.

(2) ***Open Commitments***: The children are promised that they will be kept fully informed of all aspects of their treatment.

Specifically, they will be kept informed about their therapeutic successes and failures. The children will be strongly urged to be completely forthcoming in expressing their wishes and concerns.

All the children's questions will be answered clearly, accurately and honestly.

(3) ***Final-stage Conference***: For children whose disease has progressed despite treatment.

All children six and older (unless mentally retarded) will be included, unless parents are adamantly opposed.

Children and parents will be fully informed of the course of their disease, the unavailability of any other drugs known to be effective, that cure is improbable, and that death is imminent.

The child will be told, "Most likely you will die from this disease very soon."

Children and parents will be offered two options as objectively as possible: Supportive care only (usually at home) or the use of Phase II experimental drugs. The

> Phase II drug's course of treatment and side-effects, the unlikelihood of cure, but the possibility of remission, will be clearly explained.
>
> All information will be presented to the child as objectively as possible in order not to influence his/her decision.
>
> The children will be encouraged to make their own decisions, in discussion with their parents.

For many caregivers, both professionals and parents, our first reaction might well be that this is certainly not the way we usually make such dreadfully painful, serious and difficult decisions *for* children. We might identify three major differences. First, children, even very young children, are being given the truth about their condition and treatment, even when such truths are frightening. We adults are used to protecting children from such terrible truths.

Second, children are being given truthful information so that they can make their own decisions, even the most deadly serious decisions imaginable. Normally we adults have felt it was our job, our parental duty, to bear such heavy burdens for our children, and our patients.

Finally, this model, by empowering the child to be more self-expressive and self-determinative, encourages the child's independence from his or her parents. Again, the traditional model of family unity under parental authority has not fostered such autonomy for "our" children, especially when decisions have such grave consequences. As one observer sums up the normal communication pattern in pediatric care:

> The care of children represents transactions between adults ... Children are seldom involved in the processes related to their own care.[2]

With an unusually pithy directness, Milton expresses the spirit behind the practice:

> What man in his senses would deny that there are those whom we have the best grounds for considering that we ought to deceive — as boys, madmen, the sick, the intoxicated.[3]

The same spirit that infuses this protective behavior of physicians as well as parents is rather more gracefully expressed in a passage from Chapter 40 of the Book of Isaiah:

> He will feed his flock like a shepherd. He will gather the lambs in his arms. He will carry them in his bosom, and gently lead those that are with young.

Now we need to closely examine the logic and practices of such good pediatric shepherds.

THE GOOD SHEPHERD MODEL

This traditional model is Paternalistic, Consequentialist and Conservative. It is Paternalistic, because the adult caregiver (whether familial or professional) bases restricting the child's access to the truth on the adult's judgment of what is best for the child. "Paternalism" in essence is the practice of restricting the liberty of other persons without their consent in order to better protect them from some harm, or in order to better provide them some benefit.[4]

It is Consequentialist because the "ethically" appropriate amount of truth is determined by weighing the expected consequences, harmful and beneficial, of telling and not-telling.

The rights of the child are not determinative, neither is an unqualified principle such as "Tell the Truth!" or "Do not deceive others!" As responsible therapists, the truth, like a medicine, is prescribed to children in the dosage and form calculated to do them the most good and the least harm.

Finally, this position is Conservative, which means that the principal duty for this cautious type of caregiver is to protect the child from harm. Truth is dangerous. Continuing to treat the maturing young person like a child risks less. Preserving the established parental roles gives security (at least for the adults). As a result, the burden-of-proof falls on anyone who would disrupt the traditional protective attitudes.

Examining the Shepherds' Paternalism more closely, it has a very specific logic and clear justification. Let me outline the logic of this ethical posture, and then comment briefly on each of its key components. Note the focus: Restricting another person's liberty is ethically problematic. It is in need of justification. The logic of Caregiver Paternalism provides that justification.

THE LOGIC OF CAREGIVER PATERNALISM

P-1. It is my *DUTY* to do what is necessary to foster the *BEST INTERESTS* of those in my care.

P-2. I *KNOW BETTER* than they what their best interests really are.

P-3. In order to realize their best interests, I may have to *RESTRICT THEIR RIGHTS*.

P-4. I am *BEST ABLE TO JUDGE* when their interests justify the cost of overriding their rights.

P-5. If they knew their real best interests as well as I do, *THEY WOULD APPROVE*.

When we examine this position more closely, we find that two ethical principles ground Paternalism: Duty and Beneficence.

P-1. *DUTY*: For the justified paternalist, the actions are obligatory: Shepherds must lead their sheep; Parents — and doctors — must protect their children. The rules of the role of parent or physician demand this protective commitment. Good parenting, like good caregiving is not optional. It is a matter of Duty.

BENEFICENCE: The duty is to *do good*. This seems obvious; but, the critical point is that the restrictive actions of the paternalist are justified precisely by his or her capacity to do good. One must have the intention to do good for the other person. But, one must also have the capacity to *achieve* that good. Indeed, the paternalistic justification depends on being able to do better for other persons then they can do for themselves. The Oath of Hippocrates reminds us how close this is to the heart of the matter of justifying medical practice:

> I will use treatment to help the sick according to my ability and judgment, but never with a view to injuring or wrong-doing.[5]

P-2. *SUPERIOR KNOWLEDGE*: The better the knowledge, the better the interests will be served. Therefore, whoever knows better, does better; and, whoever does better is more entitled to rule.

Paternalist must be able to claim fairly that they know better than the other person what is best for that person. For pediatric caregivers superior training and experience, logic and discipline, knowledge and understanding are used to justify that claim — and the greater power over others that then justifiably follows.

P-3. *RESTRICT RIGHTS*: The end of protecting the child's welfare justifies the means of restricting the child's freedom. The frightened child must be made to submit to essential treatment, by whatever means necessary. In some situations, liberty is not the greatest good. For the paternalists, in those situations respecting rights must yield to protecting interests.

P-4. *BEST JUDGE*: The paternalist claims the capacity to judge better than the other person when the benefits of protecting interests are sufficient to justify the costs of restricting rights. The paternalist as a Consequentialist must be able to claim superior expertise at weighing the consequences for the other, and at producing the best outcome.

P-5. *OTHER'S "APPROVAL"*: Parents, in mid-spanking, have traditionally invoked two ethical licenses: First, "I'm doing this for your own good," and Second, "When you grow up, you'll thank me." The first is obviously the justification from Benevolence. The second is more subtle. What it says is that paternalism's apparent restriction of liberty is a mistaken impression. Examine the classic term "Autonomy". Literally it means "self-ruling". To deny persons the freedom to act as they wish would seem on the face of it to violate autonomy. But, think again. In order to be *self*-ruling you must *have* a self and *be* yourself. It could be argued that a child, lacking a fully formed set of values, self-knowledge and the capacity to translate those known values into choices, does not in any meaningful way have a "self." Therefore, denying him or her freedom is not a violation of autonomy.

Consider the parallel of the intoxicated friend who wants to drive his car home. Paternalistically, you take his keys away. Have you restricted your friend's liberty? No! Just the opposite. You stopped the drunk. But, that intoxicated artifact is not your friend (hopefully), not your friend's true self. That true self would want you to stop the dangerous artifact. You could justify the present deprivation of liberty by claiming that your friend, having sobered up, will realize he was "not himself", and that you were acting as he would want you to if he were himself — and will thank you (again, hopefully).

Similarly, the Good Shepherd could claim that with children it is no offense to protect their true self, i.e., their *future mature self* with its true interests, against their current infantile artifact. As Grotius puts it,

> The first inference is that even if something which has a false significance is said to an infant or insane person no blame for falsehood attaches thereto. Quintilian, speaking of boys, said: "For their profit we employ many fictions." The reason is by no means far to seek; since infants and insane persons do not have liberty of judgment, it is impossible for wrong to be done to them in respect to such liberty.[6]

With this logical and ethical framework we can now summarize the five specific arguments that the "Good Shepherd" makes against imposing heavy truth and hard choices on children.

Arguments Against Pediatric Truth-Telling

First: Harmful! Telling "heavy" truths, no matter how well-meant, may produce severe suffering, especially in a vulnerable child. The duty of responsible caregivers is to protect their patients from pain and suffering. Remember the oft-cited first principle of medical care: *Primum non nocere*, or "Above All, Do No Harm!" To be openly told of the risks of death from a life-threatening illness, or the frightening aspects of an imminent procedure, or the smoldering dangers of a chronic illness will produce suffering. For the Good Shepherd, that creates a *prima facie* case against telling, i.e., against harming.

Note that the injunction is not "Do No Hurt!" Physicians, other caregivers, and even good parents hurt children. We pressure them and we constrain them. We threaten and punish. We subject them to unpleasant, even painful, treatments, forcefully if necessary. But, these hurts are not *harms*, if they are the necessary means to benefit the children. An immunization shot may hurt. It does not (except exceptionally) harm. What the Good Shepherd will claim is that for children, heavy truth will hurt without helping, and so produces unjustifiable harms. And, given the emotional lability and vulnerability of children, and their comparative lack of secure coping mechanisms, it is even more imperative for pediatric caregivers to use benevolent deception as preventive care.

There is another danger. Traumatized by an unmanageable truth, the child may give up hope and become non-compliant or even self-destructive. The Good Shepherd, like the good father, not only may, but must, protect his fragile, vulnerable charges from harm, including the self-inflicted harms produced if the child tries to manage dangerous truths.

Second: Useless: Adults have to face reality because they have to make real decisions. They have a need to know the full situation, including the risks of pain, suffering and death, as these are relevant to informed decision-making. Adults have the right to be fully informed because they need to be self-determining, to be "autonomous".

Children, however, are not for the most part required or permitted to make decisions about their own care. Adults, parents, and other caregivers, because they are more mature, knowledgeable and experienced, make surrogate decisions for children. On a need-to-know basis, relevant information should be imparted to parents. But, as children have no need to decide, they have no need to know.

Third: Irresponsible: Responsible caregivers for children (and other vulnerable dependents) must bear the burdens of that responsibility. The duties of adult caregivers include shielding children from threats they cannot handle and decisions they should not make. One mother of a 15 year old dying of neuroblastoma, when asked to discuss a DNR order, raced into her daughter's room and, thrusting the form at her, said, "Here, this concerns you, too. You decide!"Adults who impose such burdens on children have abdicated from their natural duties.

Fourth: Impossible: First, medical decisions are based on medical judgment. Such judgment requires a disciplined process of deliberation and a capacity to grasp an extensive body of complex information. This is hard enough for a mature, experienced, medically educated physician. It is sometimes just possible for parents. It is virtually always impossible for children. They are unable to grasp the meaning of basic factual information about disease processes and therapeutic procedures.

Second, children are ill-prepared to deliberate in a rational, realistic and responsible way about difficult choices. A meaningful choice can only be made by a fully formed self. A child's self is too inchoate, too volatile, too impressionable to be able to formulate choices as expressions of a centered set of values, of an authentic self-hood. Absent a meaningful development of self and a meaningful understanding of the options, meaningful choices are impossible.

Fifth: Unnecessary: Finally, there is no need to implant heavy truths in a child in order to discover how he or she would respond. Parents, with their innate sensitivity and extensive experience, and professionals with their disciplined awareness and educated understanding, are able to "read" the child's wishes and needs better than the child. Far from ignoring or violating the child, parents and professionals serve as responsive and responsible guardians and representatives of the child's best interests and authentic self.

In sum, the Good Shepherds, like the good parents, believe that they may, indeed at times must, deceive a child for the sake of the child. Dr. Willard Gaylin forcefully asserts this paternalistic duty,

> But there is one place where paternalism cannot be abandoned, and that is in the relationship of parent to child. Here an abandonment of parental authority would be an act of immorality, as well as a failure in nuturing. The good parent ... is expected to inhibit self-destructive impulses; he is expected to substitute his superior judgment for the short vision of the child; he is expected to use education, persuasion, seduction, and even force and coercion when necessary in the service of producing a healthy and independent adult.[7]

In sum, according to this ethical model, we may, indeed, must be Good Shepherds in order to be good parents, or good pediatric caregivers.

AUTONOMY AND PATIENT LIBERATORS

For adult ethics, the inevitable counter to a Paternalistic *Doctor* dominated relation is an autonomous *Patient* controlled relation. In a revolutionary shift of control of the Doctor-patient (or Patient-doctor) relation, Autonomy has become the ethical imperative driving the development of Informed Consent, patient refusals of treatment, Advanced Directives, and, of course, demands for Truth-Telling. Ultimately, such diverse sources as the United States Constitution's defense of individual freedom and privacy, and the philosophical opposition of John Stuart Mill and others to constraints on the individual's liberty have grounded the rights of persons to direct their own actions in accordance with their own choices based on their own sense of their own values and interests.

Increasingly over the last 30 years ago, this ethical vision of patients as autonomous individuals has come to tilt the balance of power in medical practice. Although there had been isolated cases as early at 1914, it was not until the early 1960's that the courts produced the first substantive defenses of a new requirement for physicians to secure "Informed Consent" from patients before doing invasive and/or risky things for them. Then in 1970 Professor Paul Ramsey of Princeton, published the seminal work *The Patient as Person*, in which he laid the foundations for this new advocacy of patient autonomy by applying to doctors the words of Abraham Lincoln, "No man is good enough to govern another without his consent."[8]

The Logic of Autonomy can be outlined in the same way as we laid out the Logic of Paternalism:

The Logic of Patient Autonomy

A-1. A person has the *RIGHT TO BE HIMSELF OR HERSELF.*

A-2. A person is essentially a separate, distinct *INDIVIDUAL.*

A-3. In order to be individual, a person must be autonomous, i.e., *SELF-RULING.*

A-4. In order to be self-ruling, persons must be able to *ACT* in accordance with *THEIR OWN CHOICES* based on *THEIR OWN VALUES.*

A-5. In order to so act, *OTHERS' RESPECT AND SUPPORT* are mandatory.

Examining Autonomy more closely, we find again that there are two grounding elements to its claim: The enforceable nature of *Rights*, and the essential nature of the *Individual.* Note also that as Paternalism begins with the nature of the physician, conversely Autonomy begins with the nature of the patient.

A-1. *RIGHTS*: Rights are enforceable demands, such that it would be wrong for anyone to interfere with a person exercising a right. A right, unlike a wish or desire or even a need, has a status that demands respect.[9]

A-2. The Self As *INDIVIDUAL*: Respect for persons is not all encompassing, as their wishes, needs and interests are not absolute. Superficial and peripheral wants may be sacrificed or overridden or ignored. However, respect for a person demands respect for what is essential to that person. As a cat, for example, has the right to act like a cat, so persons have the right to act as they essentially are. And the essential nature of a person is to be individual. A person is not essentially an extension or possession of anyone else. Each person is a separate distinct entity, in John Donne's charming phrase, ".... a little world made cunningly".

A-3. *SELF-RULING*: The *sine qua non* of existing as an individual is to be in control of your life, to be free. Being controlled by others, no matter how well intentioned, is a violation of the self-ruling power that is essential to being an individual. Individuality equals Autonomy.

A-4. *ACTS/CHOICES/VALUES*: Autonomy consists of acting as you choose, and choosing as you value. Only in this way can who you are be realized in what you do. And only thus can you be yourself.

A-5. *RESPECT/SUPPORT OBLIGATORY*: All individuals are dependent upon and limited by others. Freedom is fragile. Therefore, regard for the rights of others is genuine only if we give them our respect and our support. Indeed, to come full circle, as rights are enforceable demands, and as a person as Individual has the right to be autonomous, and as Autonomy can only be real if choices are supported, respect for the person's choices is obligatory.

This is the strongest argument for autonomy. It is buttressed by four other important arguments that we shall identify briefly:

(1) *Superior Knowledge*: No one experiences your life. No one else feels your feelings. No one else lives your life from the inside out. Therefore, no one knows you *as* you know yourself. Consequently, no one knows you *as well as* you know yourself. A brief personal vignette: Trying to comfort the injured eight year old, the father says, "Now, come on dear. It doesn't hurt that much." To which the child replies, "It doesn't hurt *you* that much!"

(2) *Ownership Rights*: Each person owns his or her own body. They hold title to it, and, therefore, are entitled to control it. Such ownership rights, also called "proprietary rights", authorize the owner and no one else to decide what to do with his or her private possession.

(3) *Self-Defense*: No one has the right to violate my person, my body, without my permission. Our Common Law tradition, and our traditional ethics recognize that individuals' have the right to defend themselves against unauthorized invasions of their person. Categorized as a form of "Battery", the law of Informed Consent has incorporated judgments against such non-consensual touchings.[10]

(4) *Burden of Consequences*: This is an important ethical rule-of-thumb. In general, the person who bears the burden of the consequences of a decision has the right to a say in the decision. Politically, we proclaimed "No taxation without representation." Ethically, a woman's right to make her own reproductive choices is grounded on this same moral rule.

Our next step is now clear: To draw the connection between Autonomy and Truth-telling. To be autonomous is to be able to make choices, real choices. To make such choices, the person must know what the options really are, what the real arguments are for and against each, and what the real consequences are likely to be of choosing one instead of another. A valid Informed Consent requires providing the same information.

If accurate and complete information about options is withheld, the individual will either be forced to submit blindly to others' power, or will be seduced into accepting a deceptive illusion. Without truth there can be no understanding; without understanding there can be no choice. In a word, Autonomy depends on truth-telling. Therefore, respect for autonomy demands truth-telling.

At this point, Liberators make one additional very problematic connection. They claim that the child is a person, a separate and distinct individual, and, therefore, entitled to Autonomy and to respect for his or her autonomous choices. The protective denial of truth and assertion of control by physicians, parents and other paternalistic adults is repudiated as a violation of the rights of vulnerable individuals. In a classic article, Mnookin contrasted these "kiddie libbers" with the traditional "child savers".[11] Another seminal article, also from the 1970's, described the same confrontation over attitudes towards children's rights between advocates of "Nurturance" (a.k.a. Good Shepherds) and advocates of "Self-Deliverance" (a.k.a. Liberators).[12]

While these attitudes have at times been viewed as contradictory and mutually exclusive, a more responsive and responsible view would recognize the need to balance the obligations to respect the individual person, and to protect the vulnerable child. This encompassing vision is expressed by the National Commission for the Protection of Human Subjects of Biomedical and Behavioral Research:

> Respect for persons incorporates at least two basic ethical convictions: first, that individuals should be treated as autonomous agents, and second, that persons with diminished autonomy are entitled to protection.....[13] Focusing specifically upon our responsibilities towards children, the Commission adds that "Respect for the immature .... may require protecting them as they mature."[14]

ARGUMENTS FOR PEDIATRIC TRUTH-TELLING

All responsible caregivers would recognize the need to balance respecting and protecting. Liberators are disposed to judge in many circumstances that the balance may, and indeed should be tipped more towards empowering the pediatric patient with truth and autonomy. They make five targeted objections to what they regard as the good shepherd's overly cautious protectionism. They might take as their motto the words of Justice Louis Brandeis: "The greatest danger to liberty lurks in the insidious encroachment by men of zeal, well-meaning but without understanding."[15]

First*: *NOT Harmful: Increasingly, studies indicate that withholding honest explanations from children increases their anxiety and fear. For example, a study of cancer survivors reported "lack of candor as a source of stress or other difficulty during and after the treatment period."[16]

While children, as anyone, will naturally be distressed by having to face painful procedures or frightening prognoses, we must compare that distress with the distress produced by evasion and artifice. Disclosure brings child, family and caregivers together, able to share the burdens because they share the truth. On balance, open sharing reduces the suffering, and so is less harmful.

Second*: *NOT Useless: Bluebond-Langner comments extensively on how children, who "all knew they were dying before death was imminent", were drawn into a "mutual pretense". The children had to pretend they did not know in order to protect their parents and caregivers. The children became the adults' protectors, and by so doing, sacrificed their own needs to be sick, to be dependent, to be themselves.[17] Openness helps children by letting them be themselves.

This raises another major counter to the Good Shepherd: Your attempted deception does not work. This is a very weighty point, since the major justification for benevolent deception is that it really helps the child. That can be a legitimate claim only if the deception is effective. But, careful observers report that for most children, the cover-up just does not succeed.[18] Children find out anyway, and in a worse way. Without open discussions and sharing, children's fearful fantasies create more stress and anxiety than the truth. Deception does not succeed in keeping out the fears of sickness and death. It only succeeds in keeping out the loved ones, who could have helped them deal with the fears.[19]

On the other side, numerous studies have shown how open discussion with children reduces suffering, and co-morbidity, both psychological and physiological. For example, Egbert reported on the reduction of psychological effects and post-operative complications for children who were involved in open discussions of care.[20] A study of survivors of childhood cancer found that of those informed late about their disease, 44% were well-adjusted, whereas for those informed early, 67% were well-adjusted.[21]

Of particular relevance was a survey of adolescent cancer patients and their physicians. Almost 70% of both groups agreed that more information produced less worry, not more; and over 90% of both groups agreed that more information produced more cooperative patients.[22]

Finally, we should note the absence of solid evidence to back up the Good Shepherd's fear that telling the truth will harm the patient. Aside from expressions of personal anxiety and anecdotal observations, there are, as Dr. Sanford Leiken observes, no studies that demonstrate the harmful effects of disclosure.[23]

Third*: *NOT Irresponsible: Both parents and caregivers may suffer from a conflict of interest when deciding whether or not to deal openly with a child about a painful reality. Maintaining an illusion of normality protects not only the child but also the caregivers from the burdens of having to face each other's fears and anxieties.

Chesler observes how functional deception was for both parents and staff dealing with children with cancer. By protecting children from knowledge of their illness, parents could delay their own loss of authority, continue to play the role of responsible protector, and preserve family integrity and privacy.[24] Similarly, for the staff the optimistic disguise preserved their "proper" role as the in-control, competent rescuers, appearing to fulfill their duty to protect their patient from harm.

In the judgment of Dr. Leiken,

> An overwhelming wish to protect a very sick child from disturbing information, guilt feelings, or the emotional threat posed by the imminent death of their child may overshadow parental recognition or acceptance of the juvenile's autonomy or even his or her welfare.[25]

This is well put. The problem is not that parents and physicians deliberately sacrifice a child's interests to protect their own. Rather, caring for a sick child imposes such agonizing burdens on the adults that their judgment may be skewed by their own suffering and anxiety. This suffering must be recognized and respected and dealt with — But, not at the expense of the child, not at the expense of further isolating, frustrating and frightening the child.

Fourth*: *NOT Impossible: Children do understand, oftentimes more than we realize, or want to realize. In the most substantial examination of the professional literature, Speece and Brent reviewed 40 studies of children's understanding of death.[26] They identified three components of a mature concept of death:

1. Irreversibility: There is no return.
2. Non-functionality: All living functions end.
3. Universality: Every living thing dies.

On the question of when children achieve this understanding of death, the studies reached a clear consensus. The majority of children achieve an understanding of all three components *by the age of seven!*

It should be noted that these were studies of healthy children. Many who work with sick children have been struck by the extraordinary precocity of their understanding of "adult" concerns, such as death. For example, Bluebond-Langner in her classic study of leukemic children observes how their understanding develops at an extraordinary rate, because they need to cope with extraordinary situations.[27] As a 12 year old diabetic expressed the difference between herself and her healthy peers, "They don't have to grow up as fast as I do."

From a complementary perspective, The National Commission for the Protection of Human Subjects of Biomedical and Behavioral Research has reached the same conclusion. Their report and recommendations on *Research Involving Children* concluded that:

> The Commission believes that children who are seven years of age or older are generally capable of understanding the procedures and general purpose of research and

> of indicating their wishes regarding participation. Their assent should be required in addition to parental permission.[28]

Fifth*: *NOT Unnecessary: In all humility, we should confess that we cannot always read what is going on inside a child, especially a sick child, without the help of the child. Confirmation comes from studies that compare patients and physicians perceptions of their shared experience. One study found substantial disparity between adolescent cancer patients and their physicians, with the physicians reporting significantly more patient fear, misunderstanding, discomfort, dissatisfaction and preoccupation with illness than was reported by the patients themselves.[29]

Even more important is the therapeutic benefit for the child of being respected, of being trusted with the truth. And, perhaps even more important, honest disclosure by adults fosters honest disclosure by the child. Trust engenders trust. Treating the child "like a child" takes away the need to be responsible, to be "grown-up". Involving children in understanding and dealing with serious problems may increase the children's sense of themselves as active and responsible contributors to their own care. The gifts of truth and trust may turn into therapeutic investments producing greater compliance and healthier psychological development. As Bluebond-Langner concludes,

> The issue then is not whether to tell, but how to tell, in a way that respects the children and all of their many, often conflicting needs.[30]

THE EDUCATOR MODEL

One major reason for the Shepherds' traditional reluctance to inform and empower children was due to a false dichotomy. Again, by misapplying the dominant adult model, pediatric caregivers were blinded to an age appropriate and therapeutically viable middle ground. The *Adult* Rights' model vested in the doctrine of Informed Consent created an "either/or" choice: Either the paternalistic physician ruled, or the autonomous patient ruled. (Of course, even adult doctor-patient relations are seldom so one-sided.) Believing (often correctly) that children were not prepared to handle the responsibilities and pressures of being an independent and unilateral decision-maker, the caregivers excluded them completely from honest discussions and serious decisions.

Now, let us grant that most pre-adolescent children are not capable of making major therapeutic decisions *on their own*. Few adults are, or want to. But, the consensus of developmental psychologists and developmental pediatricians is clear: Most pre-adolescent children are capable of participating in the decision-making process with their parents and caregivers.[31] They are capable of sharing the information, the understanding and the choices with their parents, their physicians and other caregiving partners. Such sharing can be both more therapeutically effective and developmentally beneficial.

Dr. William Bartholome has focused our attention on "Assent" as providing the age-appropriate and family-compatible model for pediatric care sharing.[32] The Child Assent Model, first developed by the National Commission for the Protection of Human Subjects and Biomedical and Behavioral Research in 1977, has four requirements: (1) Help the child reach an age-appropriate understanding of his or her illness, (2) Disclose the nature and, especially, the experience of all proposed interventions, (3) Examine the child's understanding, feelings and concerns and, (4) Solicit the child's expression of willingness to accept (or not) the proposed intervention.

The required role goes well beyond merely giving information and promoting compliance. The caregiver is required to be an Educator. The crucial elements are that we must seek to understand the child in his or her personal individuality — that we must try to promote the child's own understanding of himself or herself — and that we must respect that self, that person, as the child does. As Soren Kierkegaard once said, "An education is the course you run in order to catch up with yourself." The Educator's Role is to help each "student", including young persons who are ill, find his or her own way to become truly and fully himself or herself.

The fear, of course, for adults is that the empowered child will refuse to choose "correctly". But, realistically, most children are eager, sometimes too eager, to please the significant adults in their lives. When they withhold assent, it is often an important signal that there is a misunderstanding, or a fear, or a resistance to pressure that we need to hear, respect, and respond to by providing more opportunities for open negotiating.

THE PEDIATRICIAN AS EDUCATOR

The Educator's role is to foster individual growth. That, in essence, is also the Pediatrician's role. Pediatrics is a developmental specialty, as children, the focus of our attention and commitment, are developing persons. They are "in process". They are on the way to becoming bigger and stronger, more perceptive and reflective, more resourceful and independent. And, we, the pediatric caregivers, are dedicated to serving as the educators who must help them practice the skills and shape the course they must run to reach the goal of becoming autonomous adults.

Developing children's capacity for independence is declared by Leikin as children's "overriding and ultimate interest". Therefore, pediatricians have special roles, which include (1) promoting youth's mental and emotional development, (2) evaluating their degree of maturity, and (3) supporting their autonomy in decision-making when competence is reached and thus expressing respect for this person.[33]

Our responsibility is more than merely recognizing and responding to the level of capacity the maturing child has already reached. Our responsibility is to foster autonomy. As Brock put it, this commitment is to

> the aim of preparing the child with the opportunities and capacities for judgment and choice necessary for exercising self-determination as an adult.[34]

Ethically, the child has a legitimate interest in "growing-up". This creates an ethical obligation for us to provide the practice necessary to realize that essential potential.

This was the charge delivered to pediatric providers by The Sub-task Panel on Infants, Children and Adolescents of the President's Commission on Mental Health. In addition to underscoring our need to respect the individuality, privacy and autonomy of each child, they called us to involve children in decision-making as a "growing opportunity" to prepare for individual and joint decision-making in the future.[35]

Pediatric caregivers are also well aware that self-esteem is essential to child development and adult fulfillment. A basic element of secure and functional self-esteem is the belief that we have some control over persons and situations that affect us. To reinforce this belief, adults must give children the opportunity to understand the situations they are in, to make choices about those situations, and to develop their own capacities to solve the problems and cope with the pressures in those situations.[36] Pediatric Educators must teach decision-making skills to their young patients.[37] The capacity to be a good decision-maker does not mysteriously appear: it must be learned and practiced with assistance from others.[38]

To summarize: Pediatric Caregivers as Educators are able to provide tremendously important benefits by sharing truth and decision-making with children:

(1) It prepares children progressively for adult responsibilities.

(2) It increases their sense of self-esteem.

(3) It promotes their taking more personal responsibility.

(4) It increases their sense of being in control, and, therefore, increases their feelings of security.

(5) It increases their acceptance of the burdens of treatment and thus increases compliance.

Let us conclude then, with a final charge from Dr. William Bartholome:

> Children have a right to be treated as developing persons, as persons with a developing capacity for rationality, autonomy and participation in health care decision-making.[39] Given that right, and the crucial benefits for children that come from its realization, pediatric caregivers have a pre-eminent opportunity and consequent obligation to serve as Educators — providing the means, guiding the way, and supporting the efforts of children as they run the course towards becoming fully themselves.

References

1. From Nitschke, R. *et al.*, (1982). Therapeutic choices made by patients with end-stage cancer, *J. of Pediatr.*, 101, no 3, 471–476.
2. Lewis, C. E. (1983). Decision-making related to Health: When Could, Should Children Act Responsibly? In: *Children's Competence to Consent*, edited by G. B. Melton, G. P. Koocher and J. J. Saks. New York: Plenum Press.
3. quoted in Bok, S. (1978). *Lying: Moral Choice in Public and Private Life*. New York, Pantheon, p. 209.
4. Beauchamp, T. L. (1978). Paternalism. In: *Encyclopedia of Bioethics*, edited by W. T. Reich, pp. 1194–1200. New York: Free Press.
5. trans. Jones, W. H. S. (1923). *Hippocrates Vol 1*, Cambridge: Harvard U. Press.
6. Grotius, H. *On the Law of War and Peace*, Bk 3, Chapter 1, translated by F. W. Kelsey, (1925), Indianapolis: Bobbs-Merrill.

7. Gaylin, W. (1982). Competence: No Longer All or None. In *Who Speaks for the Child: The Problem of Proxy Consent*. New York: Plenum, pp. 30–31.
8. Ramsey, P. (1970). *The Patient as Person*. Princeton, NJ: Princeton University Press, p. 7.
9. Dworkin, G. (1977). *Taking Rights Seriously*. Cambridge, Mass: Harvard University Press.
10. Rozovsky, F. A. (1984). *Consent to Treatment: A Practical Guide*. Boston: Little, Brown.
11. Mnookin, R. (1978). Children's Rights: Beyond kiddie Libbers and child savers. *J. Clin. Child Psychology*, **7**:163–167.
12. Rogers, C. M and Wrightsman, L. S. (1978). Attitudes towards children's rights: nurturance or Self-deliverance. *J. Soc. Issues*, **34**:59–68.
13. National Commission for the Protection of Human Subjects of Biomedical and Behavioral Research. The Belmont Report, (1979). Washington: U.S. Government Printing Office, pp. 4–5.
14. Ibid.
15. Brandeis, L. Dissenting Opinion, Olmstead v. U.S., 277 US 438, 1928.
16. Slavin, L. A., *et al.*, (1982). Communication of the Cancer Diagnosis to Pediatric Patients: Impact on Long-Term adjustment. *Am. J. Psychiatry*, **139**(2):179–82.
17. Bluebond-Langner, M. (1978). *The Private Worlds of Dying Children*. Princeton, NJ: Princeton University Press.
18. Leiken, S., (1989). A proposal concerning decisions to forego life-sustaining treatment for young people, *J. Pediatr.,* **115**:1:17–22 and Spinetta, J. *et al.*, (1973). Anxiety in the dying child. *Pediatrics*, **56**:1034–1037.
19. Pearson, J. M. (1983). How to discuss death with patients and their families. *Consultant* pp. 85–105 and Spinetta, J., Maloney, L. (1975). Death Anxiety in the Out-patient Leukemic Child, *Pediatrics*, **56**:1034–1037.
20. Egbert, L. D., Bahit, G. E., and Welch, C. E., Reduction of post-operative pain by Encouragement and Instruction of patients: A Study of Doctor-Patient Rapport; *New England Journal of Medicine*, 1964, **270**:825–827.
21. Slavin, L. A., *et al.*, 1982 op. cit.
22. Pfefferbaum, B. *et al.*, (1982). Comparison of physicians and patients' perceptions of communications issues. *So. Med. J.*, Vol **75** No. 9, 1080–1083.
23. Leiken, S. (1983). The role of adolescents in decisions concerning their cancer therapy. *Cancer*, **71**:3342–3346.
24. Chesler, M. A. (1986). "Telling" the child with cancer: Parental choices to share information with ill children. *J. Ped. Psych.* Vol 11, No 4:497–516.
25. Leiken, S. (1989). op. cit.
26. Speece, M. W., Brent, S. B. (1984). Children's understanding of death: A review of three components of a death concept. *Child Development*, **55**:1671–1686.
27. Bluebond-Langner, M. (1978). op. cit.
28. National Commission for the Protection of Human Subjects of Biomedical and Behavioral Research (1977). Research Involving Children, DHEW, Washington: U.S. Government Printing Office, p. 16.
29. Pfefferbaum, B. *et al.*, (1982). op. cit.
30. Bluebond-Langner, M. (1978). op. cit., p. 235.
31. Bartholome, W. G. (1993). Care of the Dying Child: The Demands of Ethics, *Second Opinion* 18, no 4:25–39. cf. Melton, G. B., *et al.*, (1983). *Children's Competence to Consent.* NY: Plenum Press.
32. Bartholome, W. G. (1989). A new understanding of consent in pediatric practice. *Ped. Annals*, **18**:4:262–265.
33. Leiken S., 1989 op. cit., 18.
34. Brock, D. W. (1988). Children's competency for health care decision-making. In: *Children and Healthcare*, edited by L. Kopelman and J. Moskop. Boston, Kluwer Academic Publishers.

35. quoted in Weithorn, L. A. (1983). Involving children in decisions affecting their own welfare, in Melton, G. B., Koocher, G. P., and Saks, M. J. op. cit., p. 241.
36. Brooks, R. B. (1992). Self-esteem during school years. *Ped. Clinics of N.A.,* **39**:3:537–550.
37. King, N. M. P., Cross A. W. (1989). Children as decision-makers: Guidelines for Pediatricians. *J. Peds.*, **115**:1:10–16.
38. Lewis, C. E. (1983). op. cit.
39. Bartholome, W. G. (1989). op. cit.

6 Confidentiality and the Adolescent: An Ethical Analysis

Jeffrey Blustein

Albert Einstein College of Medicine and Mercy College, Dobbs Ferry, New York, USA

INTRODUCTION

Discussions of the principle of confidentiality and of the grounds for permissible departures from it abound in the literature of professional ethics. Most of these discussions, however, deal with confidentiality only as a feature of relationships between professionals and adults. Whether confidentiality has any distinctive value for adolescents, and what the scope of a principle of confidentiality might be when the patients or clients are adolescents is rarely considered.

The reasons for this relative neglect are perhaps not hard to appreciate. Adolescence separates childhood from adulthood and shares features of both. Neither child nor adult, the adolescent is in a process of transition psychologically, physiologically, socially, legally and ethically. Decisional capacity and maturity vary widely from early to late adolescence (approximately 11 to 20 years of age), and the extent of control parents may legitimately exercise over their children during this phase of life is unclear. Because adolescence is a transitional stage, decisions about confidentiality for adolescents are bound to be fraught with moral uncertainty, to a degree that may make similar decisions about adults seem uncomplicated by comparison.

To give some sense of the kinds of issues that arise in this area, consider the following scenarios:

Rachel is a 14-year-old high school student who has been having sexual relations with a boy she has been dating for several months. Prior to this she was not sexually active. She presents at the doctor's office with vague complaints of nausea and listlessness. To make a proper diagnosis, the physician needs to ask Rachel numerous questions, some of a sensitive nature, about her personal health behaviors. Should the physician involve her parents? Should he inform Rachel that he cannot treat her without parental involvement?

George, 16, is applying for a job as a summer camp counselor. As part of his physical, he undergoes a routine urine drug screening which comes back positive. George's parents are worried about him because his performance in school has deteriorated and he has begun to hang out with the wrong crowd. They tell the physician that they want to find out if he is taking drugs. Should the physician disclose the test result to the parents even if George doesn't want them to know?

Samantha, 15, is being treated in therapy for depression. She believes that her parents have always favored her older brother and that she has never been able to make them proud of her. In therapy she reveals that, although she has not yet attempted it, she has occasionally thought about suicide as the solution to her problems. Should the therapist tell the parents about their daughter's thoughts?

Anthony, 17, is a homosexual who lives for long stretches of time on the street, where he engages in prostitution to support himself and his drug habit. Periodically he returns home, but though his parents are concerned about him, these visits always end in quarrels and recriminations. The doctor at the outreach clinic to which Anthony goes for medical care does an HIV test, which is positive. Should the doctor inform his parents? Should he notify them before beginning treatment, or, when Anthony develops AIDS?

Each of these stories is just a sketch. Much more information about the persons involved and their circumstances would be needed before we could proceed with any degree of confidence to make ethical recommendations. Clearly, we also need a disciplined method for evaluating such information. At the end of this paper, after providing a general ethical framework for thinking about these sorts of problems, I will revisit these cases.

But, before turning to the various issues involved in confidentiality for adolescents, it is necessary to outline the psychological and moral significance of the principle of confidentiality.

THE VALUE OF CONFIDENTIALITY

Confidentiality is one of the bedrock ethical principles of the doctor–patient relationship. It is incorporated in the Hippocratic Oath and expressed in numerous contemporary medical codes of ethics. This principle, broadly construed, bars the disclosure of intimate or private information by persons to whom it has been entrusted without the authorization of the one who has revealed it.

It has wide application to a variety of professional as well as personal relationships. Physicians, psychologists, psychiatrists, and psychiatric social workers are expected (within limits) to keep the confidences of their patients, lawyers to maintain confidentiality with their clients, and priests to safeguard the privacy of the confessional. In the intimate relationships of family and friendship, the principle of confidentiality also governs, although family members and friends are typically allowed more latitude in interpreting the principle, and usually are more understanding and accepting of certain acts of noncompliance with the principle. At the heart of the concern with confidentiality in these different contexts are the fear of betrayal and exposure, whether intentional or unintentional, whether stemming from insensitivity to one's interests or from well-meaning but misguided concern — and the need for protecting oneself against such dangers.

Serious concerns are raised whenever persons reveal some aspect of themselves that to a greater or lesser degree diverges from their usual public image or identity. One may want this information kept confidential simply because one feels it is no one else's business. But, the information may also reveal personal weakness in two ways: either the information itself is about a self-perceived weakness, or its revelation to unauthorized third parties would put the individual in a vulnerable position. Particularly important are those crucial weaknesses that are closely bound up with one's self-image and identity, and information whose unauthorized dissemination would threaten the individual with serious injury or harm. Prohibitions on the disclosure of a patient's HIV status, for example, reflect this concern. Anyone who is privy to this sort of secret has enormous power over the other person. Because of this enormous power, and the potential for its abuse, whoever wants to tell his crucial secrets to another must first determine if the other can be trusted with them.

As a general rule, one will only decide to share very sensitive or potentially damaging information with another if one trusts the other to safeguard it. In professional relationships, such trust is engendered by the confidant's public acceptance of a requirement of confidentiality as binding upon his or her conduct toward the confider. In this way, the fear of betrayal is mitigated, and thereby the patient feels more secure in disclosing crucial secrets to the appropriate persons.

These remarks may help us to understand why individuals have an interest in the protections afforded by confidentiality; but, we need to go further to explain its full moral import. A confidential communication is a communication of private information. One allows or welcomes another into one's private domain on condition that what is conveyed will not be disclosed to others without one's prior authorization.

In theory, of course, privacy could exist without confidentiality, but only if one was a completely isolated, completely insulated person. In that case the rewards of intimacy, as well as the more utilitarian benefits of various professional relationships, would be unavailable. Jeffrey Reiman expresses the crucial nature of privacy:

> Privacy is a social ritual by means of which an individual's moral title to his existence is conferred.
>
> Privacy is an essential part of the complex social practice by means of which the social group recognizes and communicates to the individual that his existence is his own. And this is a precondition of personhood.[1]

Confidentiality is a significant part of this complex social practice that confers title to one's existence. The right to confidentiality is grounded in the individual's interest in being and remaining a separate and distinct person while living and sharing in the social order.

More practically, confidentiality also produces significant benefits for persons in clinical relationships. Complete candor is facilitated by the guarantee of confidentiality, and such uninhibited disclosure is necessary for accurate diagnosis and successful treatment. Without this guarantee, the patient will be selective about what he or she reveals. Since patients often are not in a position to know what the physician or therapist needs to know in order to diagnose and treat effectively, this self-censoring may jeopardize their health and welfare.

CONFIDENTIALITY AND THE DEVELOPMENTAL NEEDS OF ADOLESCENTS

To what extent are these general remarks about confidentiality applicable to the adolescent? What interests does the adolescent have in assurances of confidentiality? What is the moral significance for the adolescent of these assurances? Here we must be specific about whom the adolescent confides in, and who should be denied access to confidential information the adolescent discloses.

I take the adolescent in a more or less functional family as my point of departure. I do not mean to suggest by this any particular family structure; indeed, there is an extraordinary diversity of forms of family life in contemporary society. Rather, I refer to an ongoing relationship of supervision, support, and guidance that the adolescent has with at least one parent or parent-substitute. Admittedly rough, this characterization should be precise enough for our purposes. Later I will say something about those adolescents who lack such a relationship and who, in alarmingly increasing numbers, are presenting health care providers with new ethical quandaries.

Like adults, adolescents may choose not to share secrets with, or reveal personal information to acquaintances, teachers, employers, and so on. And, like adults, they will expect those in whom they confide not to divulge that information to others. But, of particular importance to adolescents, at least older ones, is the ability to create and enjoy a private space that excludes their *parents* or parent-substitutes, and correlatively, the secure sense that they can reveal private information to some others of their choosing without it being divulged to their parents. This is so for well-described developmental reasons.

The classic description of adolescence is that it is a phase of development characterized by the struggle to differentiate oneself from one's parents and attain independence from parental controls and judgments. The development of the individual's ego during this phase is a moving away from parents, or *individuation*, and a moving towards independent decision-making, or *autonomy*[2]. In the process of individuation, there is a sharpening of boundaries and a clarifying of the attributes of the self as distinct from those of one's parents. Adolescents come to take increasing responsibility for what they do and are, and look less to parents for validation of their choices. To accomplish this developmental task of separation from parents, the adolescent need not disavow or devalue parents and their values or attitudes. Indeed, wholesale rejection of parents often only masks an inability to separate from them in a way that adequately prepares one for adulthood. What is required, in the language of ego psychology, is that the "organization of experience be sifted through the adolescent's own increasingly differentiated ego".[3]

Two further points might also be mentioned. First, this movement toward greater autonomy is not continuous and unambivalent. Adolescents may become frightened by their newly gained independence and, feeling overextended, revert to a more dependent relationship to regain security. Second, the struggle for individuation and autonomy does not begin in later adolescence. It is an ongoing developmental task, taking different forms as the young person moves through the distinct phases of the adolescent decade.[4]

The above sketch of the basic features of adolescent development, brief as it is, helps us to understand the critical psychological role that privacy and confidentiality play in adolescence.

Among adolescents, the desire for and experience of some measure of privacy *vis-à-vis* parents, and for confidentiality in communicating with others are essential parts of the individuation process. Adolescents who are denied these opportunities typically experience feelings of incompetence and suffer a lack of self-esteem. Parents and other adults who, through ill-will or misunderstanding, do not respect adolescents' needs for privacy and confidentiality, risk doing them serious harm by hindering the progressive development of self-differentiation.

Among adolescents, privacy and confidentiality play a critical developmental role. Their moral import must be understood accordingly. In this transitional stage, the rights to privacy and confidentiality are not grounded on having achieved the moral status of an autonomous decision-maker. Rather, they serve principally to protect the adolescent's fundamental interest in developing into an autonomous agent, into an adult individual. Adolescents must first gain difference and distance from internalized parents if they are later to have a life of their own, and they must practice having the rights to privacy and confidentiality as adolescents if they are to take full advantage of these rights as adults. In short, a basis for a distinctively adolescent right to privacy and confidentiality can be found in the psychological requirements for becoming an independent, self-sufficient adult. Adolescents are particularly anxious about disclosure of secrets to their parents, whom they may regard as having often intruded in their private lives. Adolescents' essential developmental need to outgrow being their parents' "child", should reinforce the caregiver's commitment to protecting their privacy, especially from their parents.

Still, adolescents, while no longer children, are not yet adults; and the specific contours of adolescent rights to privacy and confidentiality are affected by this transitional status. To some extent, adolescents are legitimately subject to adult supervision and guidance — specifically, to *parental* supervision and guidance if the adolescent is part of a functioning family — and they have not completely outgrown the dependency needs of childhood. What then is the scope of the adolescent's right to confidentiality? When should exceptions be made and confidentiality be breached?

SETTING LIMITS: MATURITY AND HARM TO SELF

When should the adolescent's confidant, for example, a psycho-therapist or physician, break confidentiality and reveal private information to a parent? The answer depends on a number of factors: the maturity of the adolescent, the potential for harm to self or others of the adolescent's behavior and choices, and the ethical grounding of parental involvement in adolescent decision-making. Let us begin with the issue of maturity.

Setting aside the obvious and important fact that maturity varies a good deal from one adolescent to another, what might be meant by saying that an adolescent is "immature"? In part, this reflects a judgment about the status of adolescent concerns, interests, values, and goals, made from the vantage point of adulthood. The judgment I am referring to is not a condescending one, or at least not entirely condescending. It is acknowledged that the sorts of things adolescents typically care about — parental disapproval, peer acceptance, dating, idealistic causes, etc. — matter a great deal to them and should not be trivialized. It is also conceded that these concerns do have their appropriate place and value for an adolescent.[5]

Nevertheless, in calling the adolescent "immature", we (adults) are expressing the belief that these admittedly age-appropriate choices and concerns, and the behaviors that embody them, are not to be taken fully seriously. Perhaps they are means to what will be taken more seriously in adult life; perhaps we just do not regard them as making a significant contribution to the overall value of one's life. Adults not uncommonly say, for example: "If I knew then what I know now, those things that mattered so much to me as an adolescent would not have consumed so much of my time and energy, and I would have acted differently." And so, one thing that might be meant by saying adolescents are immature is just that they have not attained the perspective needed to properly evaluate the enduring significance of many of their immediate concerns.

The fact that an adolescent may care about certain things out of proportion to their value as judged from the privileged perspective of adulthood is a function of the limited nature of his life experience. But decisions he makes in pursuit of his objectives may nevertheless exhibit a degree of intelligence, rationality, and perceptiveness that is quite adult-like. It might be the case, in other words, that an adolescent deals with his immature concerns in a mature manner.

A second way of construing "immaturity" has to do not with the character of adolescent concerns and values, but rather with their intellectual, volitional, and emotional capacities. For example, maturity is defined in part in terms of the possession of a cluster of related cognitive and reasoning skills: the ability to consider possibilities that are not immediately present, to entertain alternative courses of action simultaneously and compare them in terms of short- and long-term consequences, to plan ahead in order to achieve successful outcomes, and to engage in second-order thinking about one's thoughts and inner states. In addition, the mature individual must be able to utilize knowledge in a manner attuned to the particular situation he is in and to regulate his conduct in accordance with his deliberative judgments. Other elements of maturity include the ability to control the expression of impulses, to rely on one's self rather than on external forces, events, or authorities to solve problems, and the capacity to empathize with the perspective of others.[6]

Maturity here is a matter of possessing these and other psychological capacities deemed necessary for mature decision-making, and typically adolescents possess them to some degree. Does this mean that maturity itself should be thought of as something that is possessed in different degrees? Or should we think of it rather as a threshold concept that divides people into those who are and those who are not mature? The answers depend on what we take to be the function of judgments of maturity. If their function is like that of competency determinations, if, that is, an ascription of maturity means that a person's decisions should not be overridden by others, then maturity, like competence, is a threshold concept.

If we regard maturity as a threshold concept, there are two ways of describing the threshold. The threshold may be more or less fixed: for all types of decisions, the level of attainment of the above capacities that is required for maturity is the same. Most adolescents in their early and middle teens would probably fall below the required level, many more adolescents in their late teens and most adults would probably fall above it. Alternatively, and this is the construal I prefer, the threshold might fluctuate depending on the nature and consequences of the decision that is being made. As the interests at stake for the individual become more consequential, the threshold of maturity would be raised. Specifically with respect to adolescents, the question would not be, "Is this adolescent mature, according to some fixed standard of maturity?" rather, it would be, "Does this adolescent have the maturity that is adequate to make this (sort of) decision?" Since maturity is now decision-relative, an adolescent may have the requisite maturity to make some decisions but not others.

An example will help clarify different senses of immaturity as applied to adolescents. One of the striking characteristics of this time of life is the adolescent's penchant for exploration and experimentation combined with a sense of his or her own invulnerability. Adolescents have not yet attained full adulthood, and they prepare for it by, in a very real sense, playing at being adult. Not yet at the stage of life when they have to assume adult responsibilities and make hard choices about what they are going to do with their lives, they explore different life possibilities, different identity alternatives, trying each on for size, as it were. (This fact about adolescence, it should be noted, is not independent of culture. In simpler societies than ours, adolescents have little freedom of choice with respect to their life paths.) And they do this with a fervor and inconstancy that adults often find bewildering. David Norton describes this aspect of adolescence eloquently:

> The intensity of adolescence's investment in each new possibility is likewise functional, for what it must explore is lifetimes, yet it does not have a bundle of life-times at its disposal. Therefore, it requires successive "cram-courses" in which intensity substitutes for duration. By participatory enactment, adolescence in a week traverses the course of a lifetime.[7]

Facilitating this process is the adolescent's failure to recognize or appreciate the potential seriousness of many of his or her choices. Indeed, the exploration of life options would be seriously hampered if adolescents were as risk-averse as adults normally are.

Taking risks is inherent in adolescence, and to some extent risk-courting behavior, given its developmental role, is age-appropriate. Adults may not attach the same value to thrill-seeking that adolescents do and may label the extremism of adolescence immature. But, adults ought to be tolerant of it (within limits), because adolescents cannot complete the work of adolescence if they are not given the freedom to explore and take risks that adults might eschew.

Not all risk-taking behavior is on a par, however. The risk to the adolescent of smoking, for example, is less serious in the short run than the risk of playing "chicken" with high-powered automobiles; the risks of walking around at night in somewhat unsafe areas of New York City accompanied by only a few friends are not equivalent to the risks associated with unprotected promiscuous sex. Referring back to the decision-relative threshold conception of maturity, it is reasonable to argue that as the likelihood and severity of the potential harm to the adolescent increase, the threshold should be raised. It may rise to such a level, in fact, that few adolescents of a certain age will be deemed mature enough to make a particular sort of decision. In other words, there may be some risks that the adolescent does not have the maturity to take, and from which, therefore, he or she should be protected.

I believe there are such risks and that one factor to consider in delineating the scope of the adolescent's right to confidentiality is the dangerousness to the adolescent of his or her actual or intended conduct. It would be morally irresponsible for a health care professional to promise an adolescent, or an adult for that matter, to keep confidential everything he or she reveals during the course of their relationship. The professional should make it clear to the adolescent at the outset that confidentiality will not necessarily protect the adolescent from having information about dangerous behavior revealed to others (e.g., parents), and examples should be provided to illustrate the sort of behavior that might trigger a breach of confidentiality. At the same time, the professional should let the adolescent know that revelations of actual or intended dangerous behavior will not automatically lead to outside involvement. Other possibilities, short of actually breaking confidentiality, should be exhausted first, and the adolescent should be told that every reasonable effort will be made to maintain confidentiality.

While the health care professional should reserve the right to divulge confidential information in these situations, there is normally much that is revealed in the professional–adolescent patient relationship that is of a more "innocent" nature and that does not or should not raise concerns about dangerousness to self. A confidential relationship of this sort gives the adolescent an opportunity to share perceptions and feelings — of joy, shame, loneliness, anxiety, etc. — that he or she might be acutely uncomfortable sharing with friends and especially parents. Often these feelings have to be expressed and worked through apart from parents, because they arise out of the adolescent's attempt to separate, psychologically, from them. As we might say, sometimes an adolescent just needs a sympathetic adult to talk to, someone other than his or her parents, because even if they are generally supportive and caring, they are also part of the problem.

How a physician, say, reacts to revelations by a patient of behavior that is dangerous to self may vary, and justifiably so, depending on whether the patient is an adolescent or an adult. What might lead the physician only to remonstrate with the adult patient, might, with the adolescent, lead the doctor to turn to outsiders for help.

What can justify this different response? Part of the answer, as was said earlier, has to do with the discrepancy between the possible impact of certain risky or injurious choices on the individual's life and the typical adolescent's tenuous grasp of the future. Some choices are so serious as to be life-threatening; some choices, while perhaps not life-threatening, pose a risk of long-term and far-reaching deleterious consequences for the life the individual will lead. Yet the normal adolescent, unlike the normal adult, lives very much in the here and now; reality is felt to be reversible and a sense of permanency is lacking. This mismatch between the seriousness of their actions and the narrowness of their vision, between the likelihood and severity of bad outcomes and the adolescent's appreciation of these risks, creates an opening for more permissible breaches of adolescent confidentiality.

This is not to say that therapists or physicians should never divulge confidential information about adult self-destructive or dangerous behavior. Indeed, in some instances (e.g. heavy use of drugs or alcohol), attempts at persuasion may not be sufficient, morally speaking. But there may still be a difference here that is important for the practicing professional: *when* confidentiality is appropriately breached may be affected by whether the patient who is a danger to him or herself is an adult or an adolescent. Adults can often be trusted to return for follow-up, whereas adolescents often cannot, and the professional may decide that he cannot let much time elapse before alerting others to the fact that the adolescent patient is in danger of harming him or herself.

THE PROS AND CONS OF PARENTAL INVOLVEMENT

Developmental maturity and the risk of harm to self (and others) are factors to consider in deciding when and whether adolescent confidentiality should be maintained. But, even if there is reason to believe that confidentiality should not be maintained in a particular case, there is a further question about the adults to whom the confidential information should be disclosed. Specifically, on what grounds can informing the adolescent's parents be justified?

There are two ways of attempting to justify parental involvement, even if the adolescent desires confidentiality: their *right* to know, and the *benefits* of their knowing. First, parents have a right to know about critical decisions that may have long-lasting and far-reaching consequences for their adolescent's well-being because they are generally assumed to be loving and concerned caretakers who try to do what is best for their child, and because, as parents, society grants them a wide latitude to structure family life as they see fit.[8]

If parents generally have a right to know, defined and grounded in this way, then they ought to be notified of their adolescent's critical decisions unless there is compelling reason not to do so. In other words, there is a moral presumption — albeit a rebuttable one — in favor of parental notification.

Another argument for such a presumptive right to know applies only to those adolescents whose care is covered by their parents' insurance or personal funds. Since in these cases the parents are paying for their adolescent's health care, the reasoning goes, the parents have a correlative right to at least be notified before such care is provided, unless there is compelling reason not to do so. "I have a right to know what I'm paying for," a parent may say. Indeed, the parent may go further: "Since I'm paying for it, my consent is necessary". Furthermore, besides financial concerns, parents may be seriously affected by their adolescent's actions. As the bearers of the burdens of the consequences of their children's secrets, they may claim the right to be aware.

The second justification for parental involvement looks only to the benefits for the adolescent of parental disclosure. The argument here is not that parents have some *prima facie* right to know that grounds a presumption in favor of parental notification. Rather, the presumption runs the other way: maintain adolescent confidentiality until there is a compelling reason *not* to do so. The physician would have to make a careful examination of each case, weighing the consequences, good and bad, for the adolescent, of telling and of not telling. A decision to notify would only be justified if convincingly shown to be the best way to help protect the adolescent from the consequences of his or her immaturity, consequences that are deemed serious enough to warrant adult involvement and to justify the "harms" of breaching confidentiality.[9]

Whether there should be a presumption in favor of parental notification or a presumption in favor of adolescent confidentiality would seem to depend in part on the age of the adolescent. Since the maturity to make one's own health care decisions occurs with greater frequency among older than younger adolescents, a stronger case can be made for the latter presumption among older adolescents than among younger ones.

Even for some younger adolescents there might be circumstances in which there should not be a presumption in favor of parental notification. If parents are totally uninvolved in the young person's life and provide no support or supervision, then they are parents in name only and have no presumptive right to be involved in his or her medical care. Nevertheless, these adolescents will normally still need to consult with and receive emotional support from some trusted adult.

The presumption in favor of parental disclosure can be overturned if parental involvement might itself cause serious risks for the adolescent. Even when the adolescent lacks the maturity to reach a sound decision on his or her own, parental involvement in this particular instance might be more damaging than helpful to the adolescent, and hence unwarranted.

In addition, it is unjustified to argue that parents have an unqualified right to be informed about all the tests and treatments their adolescent is receiving because they are paying for the adolescent's health care. Indeed, there might be a compelling reason to maintain confidentiality despite this fact. As a practical matter, however, it might be difficult to do so if parents are paying the bills. While the parents' insurance carrier can usually be billed for an office visit without revealing to them the confidential nature of the visit, confidentiality may be a barrier to payment for lab tests. In this case, if the adolescent cannot pay for the tests himself, the physician might either offer him a reduced rate or refer him to an agency that charges on a sliding scale.

How can a physician tell whether parental involvement would threaten the adolescent's well-being? Should the physician rely on the adolescent's own assessment of the benefits and risks of parental involvement? The problem here concerns the accuracy of the adolescent's perception of the likely consequences of parental involvement. Particularly when adolescents seek medical care for sensitive problems like sexually transmitted diseases or drug abuse or pregnancy, they may be extremely reluctant to involve their parents and might very well both exaggerate the degree of adverse parental response to their predicament and underestimate the support their parents can provide. When adolescents do resist parental involvement, physicians should try to ensure that this reluctance is not based on such misperceptions. Unless there is clear evidence that parental involvement would be more hurtful than helpful to the adolescent, physicians should at least encourage adolescents to involve their parents in their medical care.

In general, an adolescent's reluctance to involve his or her parents ought to be taken seriously, especially if it persists despite attempts to explain how parental involvement can be beneficial. But, of course, parents are not the only adults who could offer advice and counsel. Friends, relatives, teachers, clergy, etc. might be available instead, and physicians should urge their adolescent patients to consult with them. But, what if the adolescent resists all adult involvement, involvement that the physician believes would be helpful for him or her? Or what if no parents or parent substitutes are available? Should the physician refuse to treat under these conditions? To answer this question, the physician should consider whether the adolescent will then in fact not receive treatment, and if so, whether he or she faces greater harm by not receiving treatment or by receiving treatment with only the benefit of the adult physician's involvement. Presumably there will be some situations in which the risks that attend the lack of treatment outweigh the risks that attend treatment without a familial adult. In such circumstances, physicians' therapeutic duty would oblige them to accept this additional responsibility and treat the otherwise unsupported adolescent.

ADOLESCENT CONFIDENTIALITY AND THE LAW

Ordinarily, the consent of a parent is required for the medical treatment of a minor child. However, by common-law tradition, and in some states by statute, two categories of adolescents are legally authorized to consent to their own medical care: the *Mature Minor* and the *Emancipated Minor*. Mature Minors are persons under the age of 18, and usually over 15 years, who are judged to possess the capacity for giving informed consent (assessed by maturity, intelligence, and ability to make reasoned decisions). Emancipated minors are youngsters who are married, serving in the armed forces, living apart from their parents and managing their own financial affairs, or who otherwise demonstrate clear patterns of independent living. In addition to laws which authorize minors who have attained a particular status to give their own consent for medical services, every state has some statutes that permit minors to consent to medical care for particular health problems. The services for which minors are most commonly permitted to give their own consent are pregnancy-related care (including contraceptive services), diagnosis and treatment of sexually transmitted or contagious diseases (including, in some states, AIDS or HIV infection), alcohol and drug treatment, and outpatient mental health counseling.

Legal provisions that authorize minors to consent to their own care do not automatically protect the confidentiality of that care, however. Some state laws provide that when the minor has a right to consent to care, disclosure is allowed only if the minor gives his or her permission; others state explicitly that parents may not be informed over the objections of the minor. Other state laws permit health care professionals to notify parents over the objections of their minor child, or grant parents access to their minor child's medical records, without addressing the potential for conflict with the minor's wishes. State laws regarding confidentiality of adolescent health care thus vary considerably among states.[10]

The laws regarding adolescent confidentiality are an important part of the context within which health care professionals practice, and they should familiarize themselves with the specific provisions that apply in their states. But, many of the questions physicians and other health care providers face when providing health care to adolescents are ethical in nature, and knowledge of the law cannot answer these. In some cases, the law itself leaves room for the exercise of moral judgment: laws may only permit parental notification, thus providing latitude to the health care professional to disclose or not. And even when the law creates an obligation not to breach confidentiality, it might still be resisted if the professional feels strongly enough that this is the morally proper thing to do in the particular case and is willing to risk legal liability for his or her actions.

CARING FOR THE UNSUPERVISED ADOLESCENT

My discussion of adolescent confidentiality has been geared to those adolescents who come from more or less intact families. But in the real world of adolescent health care there are many adolescents who do not fit this description. No discussion of adolescent confidentiality can be complete without at least a brief mention of the unsupervised or functionally alone adolescents, those who do not have an ongoing relationship of supervision, support, and guidance with a parent or adult. Some of these adolescents are living at home with parents who are unwilling or unable to care for and supervise them; some have been orphaned by the early death of parents; some are runaways, "throwaways", street kids, or other "out-of-home" youths who are at high risk for medical and psychological problems of various sorts. Increasingly, pediatricians, adolescent medicine specialists, and primary care physicians are caring for such adolescents and confronting new and complex ethical (as well as legal) problems as a result.

The psychological portrait of unsupervised adolescents probably deviates in important ways from the account of normal adolescence presented above. The fact of being unsupervised can have a major impact on the development of the different components of maturity, and the effects are likely to vary depending on the reason for the lack of adult supervision. Street kids, for example, may seem to be more mature than their counterparts who live at home under firm parental guidance. But, what seems to be maturity may actually only be a kind of superficial and shrewd adaptation to the hazards of their precarious existence. In addition, I noted earlier that risk-taking is to some extent an inherent feature of normal adolescence. Among street kids, runaways, and the like, however, risk-courting behavior is typically more extreme, as fears of danger are overwhelmed by more immediate needs for food, shelter, care, and money to support themselves. Health care professionals may thus find themselves dealing with youngsters who live in a significantly more dangerous world, who pose a greater risk of harm to themselves than so-called normal adolescents, and who, at the same time, have no parent or other adult in their lives who is able to provide them with support and guidance.

Involving parents in the medical or psychological care of these adolescents, either with or without the patient's concurrence, may be neither feasible nor desirable. Indeed, a requirement of parental involvement may deter a significant number of these adolescents from seeking needed care at all. And yet these adolescents, because of their peculiar vulnerability and because they are thrust into a world for which they may not be psychologically prepared, have a special need for some adult protection and support. The problem for the health care professional and for society as a whole is how to ensure that they get this protection and support without depriving them of necessary medical or mental health services.

PROBLEM CASES

I will close with some brief comments about the four cases described at the beginning of this paper.

Samantha: It is not ethically acceptable for a physician to shield a suicidal patient like Samantha behind a wall of confidentiality. Though her psychiatric problems may stem from her relationship with her parents, this is not by itself a reason to exclude them from notice of her potentially lethal behavior. The parents should be informed and should be encouraged to seek psychiatric help along with their daughter.

George: The 16-year-old who does not want his parents to know that he has tested positive for drugs, is a different story. A positive test result is not by itself conclusive proof of an adolescent at high risk from substance abuse. If George is in fact a user, the best method for detecting this is candid discussion in which specific questions about drug use are part of an overall psychosocial history. Informing George's parents of the test result is likely to establish an adversarial relationship between George and his physician rather than a therapeutic one and to create conflicts between George and his parents that will exacerbate his problems.

Rachel: This young woman might not want her parents to know that she has been having sexual relations with her boyfriend. She may fear that her parents will be angry and rejecting if they find out. Perhaps she is wrong about this: but, in any case, she will not be forthcoming with the physician about her sexual behavior if she knows that he will inform her parents. If she is found to be pregnant, she may want to carry the pregnancy to term or have an abortion. Either option carries risks, physical as well as emotional; and Rachel, at 14, may lack the maturity and judgment to reach a sound decision on her own. Still, the physician should not inform the parents against her wishes, for ultimately it is Rachel, not the physician, who is the one to decide whether, on balance, parental involvement is advisable. The physician should, however, encourage Rachel to discuss her pregnancy with her parents, and should encourage her to consult other adults who can give her support and guidance during this crisis if her parents are not to be involved.

Anthony: For this homosexual youngster who is estranged from his parents, confidentiality *vis-à-vis* his parents has probably been necessary for his getting whatever testing and medical treatment he has received while living on the street. Health care professionals have good reasons to be concerned about losing street kids to follow-up, and any breach of confidentiality is likely to undermine the fragile trust that providers have managed to build up with their patients. Nevertheless, it is important for providers to attempt to link Anthony up with some adult, whether a relative, friend, or care provider, who can help him deal with the crisis of learning he is infected with HIV, and, later on, with the challenges of coping with AIDS.

Acknowledgments

I want to thank Dr. Norman Brier and his colleagues at the Rose Kennedy Center for Research in Mental Retardation and Human Development for sharing with me some of their insights as practising psychiatrists into problems of adolescent confidentiality, and Dr. Alan Fleischman for a number of helpful comments on an earlier draft of this paper.

References

1. Privacy, Intimacy, and Personhood. In *Today's Moral Problems*, second edition. R. Wasserstrom (Ed.). New York: Macmillan Publishing Co. 1979, p. 387.
2. For a discussion of individuation and autonomy, see the following: Ruthellen Josselson (1980). Ego Development in Adolescence. In *Handbook of Adolescent Psychology* Joseph Adelson (Ed.). New York: John Wiley and Sons. pp. 190–197; Richard A. Gardner (1988). *Psychotherapy with Adolescents* Cresskill, New Jersey: Creative Therapeutics. pp. 30–42; *Normal Adolescence: Its Dynamic and Impact* New York: Group for the Advancement of Psychiatry. 1968, pp. 795–816; Irene M. Josselyn (1952) *The Adolescent and His World* New York: Family Service Association of America. pp. 47–55. Dr. Gardner's book also contains a helpful discussion of confidentiality in child, adult, and adolescent therapy, pp. 437–449.

3. Josselson (1980). ibid., p. 192.
4. See Josselson (1980), and *Normal Adolescence*, op. cit.
5. For a philosophical discussion of the notion of period-relative goods, see Michael Slote (1983). *Goods and Virtues* Oxford: Clarendon Press. pp. 13–22. Slote develops this notion as part of a larger philosophical investigation of human virtue and personal good.
6. See Daniel Keating (1980). Thinking Processes in Adolescence. In: *Handbook of Adolescent Psychology*, Joseph Adelson (Ed.). New York: John Wiley and Sons. pp. 212–220; and D. W. Brock (1989). Children's Competence for Health Care Decision-making. In: *Children and Health Care: Moral and Social Issues* Kluwer Academic Publishers. I have also drawn here from Dr. Norman Brier's Hunter Lecture, delivered at Montefiore Medical Center, Bronx, New York, 2 December, 1992.
7. Norton, D. (1976). *Personal Destinies*. Princeton: Princeton University Press. p. 183.
8. For more on parents' rights, see my On the Doctrine of *Parens Patriae*: Fiduciary Obligations and State Power. *Criminal Justice Ethics,* **2**(2) (Summer/Fall 1983): 39–47.
9. The two presumptions are distinguished in R. S. Moore and A. Hofmann (Eds.) (1982). *American Academy of Pediatrics Conference on Consent and Confidentiality in Adolescent Health Care.* American Academy of Pediatrics. pp. 21–22.
10. This review of law is drawn from Abigail English (1990). Treating Adolescents: Legal and Ethical Considerations. *Medical Clinics of North America,* **74**(5):1097–1112.

7 Ethical Issues in General Pediatric Practice

Andrew P. Mezey

Professor of Pediatrics, Albert Einstein College of Medicine

INTRODUCTION

Pediatricians engaged in the general practice of pediatrics have numerous interactions with children and their parents in the course of a day. Some involve, or should be perceived as involving, ethical dilemmas. However, most pediatricians in general practice have had little or no formal training in bioethics.

In preparing to write this chapter I interviewed a number of pediatricians in general private practice. Some interviews were done individually, either in person or over the telephone; others were in informal groups at conferences. It was not a random selection; all were well-known to me, they were all trained in major academic centers, all were graduates of American medical schools, all were white males except one, all were in small group practices in suburban, relatively affluent settings, and none had formal training in bioethics, though one had taken a bioethics course in medical school. They were, however, thoughtful individuals, had kept current in pediatrics and regularly attended continuing education courses. Though they lacked formal training in bioethics, and tended not to think of what they did using the specific criterion of whether it seemed "ethical" or not, these pediatricians did use an "ethical" construct in reaching decisions, perhaps because they had been trained to think clearly about what they did and why they did it. This chapter explores the areas of general pediatric practice that, at some level, require an appreciation for and an understanding of ethical issues. This chapter also details what actually happens in several actual general pediatric practices, with my personal comment by the author. I believe that what is detailed is representative of the current practice of general pediatrics in private middle class settings.

The chapter is divided into three sections, separating the ethical issues facing pediatricians into three broad categories:

1. Physician-industry relationships.

2. Physician-patient/family relationships.

3. Physician-health insurer relationships.

The AMA has developed guidelines to help their members assess how they should act when accepting "gifts" from industry.[1] The AAP has adopted the AMA guidelines and is working on its own set. Also of concern to the AAP has been the issue of pediatricians selling prescription drugs in their offices.[2] These two issues, acceptance of gifts and physicians acting as pharmacists, have implications for what kind of treatment, what brand of treatment, how much treatment and at what cost, a patient will receive.

The direct relationship between the pediatrician and the patient and family creates ethical issues of confidentiality, especially as they relate to adolescent sexuality and drug usage, issues of suspected child abuse or neglect, issues of child custody, and issues of conflict between the pediatrician and the parent, usually regarding treatment decisions or acceptance of a diagnosis such as mental retardation.

Lastly, the third area posing real and potential ethical problems is the area of access and quality. This takes two general forms: how to deal with the family who cannot afford medical care or who has Medicaid- a form of insurance which, in most states, pays only a fraction of the physician's usual fee; and how to interact with insurance companies who "manage care", who, thereby, effectively limit the ability of the pediatrician to choose the site of, the kind of, and the amount of treatment. This last issue, the "management" of care, elicited the most passion from the pediatricians interviewed.

PEDIATRICIAN-INDUSTRY RELATIONSHIPS

Gifts From Industry

The American Academy of Pediatrics has adopted the American Medical Association's guidelines regarding gifts from industry. In essence, both the AMA and the AAP believe that industry-physician interactions are divided into 3 major types: 1. Product promotion to individuals by advertising, personal detailing and provision of samples; 2. Company promotion by provision to individuals and groups of non-educational gifts, parties, trips and services; and 3. Company promotion to individuals and groups, including hospitals, medical schools and professional societies, through the support of educational activities, research grants and contracts, professional awards, development funds and publication subsidies.[1]

Pediatricians in general practice relate mainly to the first type- the interaction with the "detail man", or woman, who visits at the beginning or end of office hours, leaving samples of medications, formula, growth charts, and brochures. Our group of pediatricians saw this activity as being of benefit to patients rather than to themselves. For the most part, the samples are given to patients as starter doses. An example often mentioned by the pediatricians interviewed was giving a free sample of an antibiotic to a patient while awaiting the results of a throat or urine culture. An example of formula sample use was in the course of treating someone with diarrhea who needed to be started on a soy-based formula. Being able to give a formula sample in the office is convenient for the parent. Growth charts supplied by pharmaceutical houses are perceived as acceptable by pediatricians, having experienced this practice in their residency training. Brochures produced by drug companies are judged to be well-written and accurate, and not thought of by pediatricians as a form of advertising, since the choice of the type of product given to the infant is usually made by the pediatrician rather than by the parent reading a brochure.

It is true that experience with new antibiotics, typically the broad spectrum oral cephalosporins, are introduced by the detail man to the pediatrician through the office use of these samples. It is also true that the drug companies hold patents on these medications and they are thus much more expensive than the older antibiotics. On the other hand, the pediatricians interviewed, to a person, stated that they chose the most appropriate antibiotic for the specific situation. A child whom they thought should be treated with amoxicillin for otitis media received amoxicillin. The samples were used when a beta-lactamase resistant antibiotic was judged to be indicated or when there was a compliance problem, requiring the use of a medication that could be given only once per day. Thus, although many others have expressed concerns, none of the pediatricians surveyed felt that there was a potential or real conflict or ethical problem in this type of industry-physician interaction.

Clearly, the pharmaceutical houses believe that there is value in employing individuals to visit pediatricians in their offices and to offer them free samples of medications, formula, brochures, and growth charts. In North America and Great Britain over one third of the industry's promotional budget is allotted to detailing and there is approximately one pharmaceutical representative for every 15 physicians.[2] The value to the industry is the promotion of their products in the pediatrician's office, a place that consumers view as an ethical and friendly haven. The drug companies believe that the visibility of their brand name in this setting will lead to increased sales of their products.

However, the pediatricians did *not* see the promotion of products in their offices as directly influencing their own choice of a product. Their arguments went as follows: For this patient I must use an antibiotic that is resistant to the effects of beta-lactamase. Why shouldn't I use a sample of something I have in the office? If I didn't have that sample I would use another antibiotic of its type in any case. The sample given to me by the detail man costs the patient nothing. It allows me to gain experience with a new medication that may be better than what is now available to me. For me the issue is not the particular brand but the type of medication needed for effective treatment of the patient; and that is in no way affected by having samples of the right type in the office.

In these cases the patient benefits, but so does the pharmaceutical company. The next time the child has an ear infection, and if the sample previously used effected a cure, the parent may very well ask the doctor to prescribe that brand. If the child gets diarrhea again and needs a soy formula, it is likely that the brand that was given as a sample will be selected. In both instances the drug company has increased its sales by using the pediatrician's office as an advertising vehicle. The pediatricians interviewed argued that this is reasonable since, for the most part, the choice of the brand of antibiotic or the brand of soy formula is neutral to them. If, at a later date, the parents prefer one brand over another because of a previous experience, that is the parents' choice. This is consistent with the culture in the United States; in a market economy we have a choice of different brands of similar products. Thus, parental preference of a formula or an antibiotic by brand name based on prior experience is consistent with normal patterns of consumer behavior.

However, this apparently innocuous cooperation between physicians and drug companies has very forceful critics. Dr. Lewis Margolis of the University of North Carolina asserts that accepting such favors violates the fundamental duties of the physician. The companies spend between $5,000 and $8,000 per physician on marketing strategies because they have documented to their satisfaction that it does change prescribing behavior. And those added costs ultimately are paid for by patients, who often can ill afford expensive medication. Most important for Dr. Margolis, it creates a clear conflict of interest, as the physicians traditional role as exclusively the *patient's* advocate, now is compromised by also serving as the *company's* advocate. He concludes:

> The belief by physicians that they can remain objective in the face of marketing efforts is likely to be a manifestation of the self-deception to which professionals, in their search for autonomy, are susceptible.[3]

It seems to me that the practice that the pediatricians follow agrees with the AMA guidelines for gifts from industry. The benefits of giving families samples of medication or formula and of the pediatrician using the educational literature and growth charts developed by a pharmaceutical company appears, by reasonable argument, to outweigh the effects of any bias that may occur. In these instances, the belief of practicing pediatricians that acceptance of "gifts" does not compromise their ability to treat the patient properly rings true to me.

In my own general pediatric practice and, later, as the director of a pediatric service in an academic center, I had frequent contact with agents of pharmaceutical houses. As I think back on my own prescribing habits and the detail men and women I have known, I am not aware that I have been influenced, *in the long run*, by the gifts of pens and scratch pads and the samples of growth charts, formula, cough and cold preparations, antibiotics, or even the sponsorship of lectures and lunches for house staff. I use amoxicillin as my first line medication for otitis media; in my area it still works as well as it did 15 years ago and I do not prescribe antihistamine-decongestant preparations for otitis media. I do not look at the name of the company that printed the growth charts; I assume them to be reasonably accurate. I advocate breast feeding and have no formula preference if the mother does not wish to breast feed or wishes to discontinue breast feeding. I cannot remember the last time I prescribed a soy formula for one of my patients after an episode of diarrhea. On teaching rounds or in my lectures on the management of gastroenteritis, I do advocate the use of soy formula in certain situations, but not by brand name. And I believe my habits are not very dissimilar from those of the majority of pediatricians currently in practice in the United States.

I do believe, however, that in the short term, the efforts of pharmaceutical companies to influence the prescribing habits of physicians are very successful. Someone comes along and says "Try this, your patients will love it". The product is made by a reputable firm and it has been approved for distribution by the Food and Drug Administration (FDA). You try it, despite the fact that you have not read about it in the literature. This scenario is a common one, particularly when a medication is first introduced and when its price is high. This, however, is not an appropriate way to practice medicine. One ought to spend the time looking up the articles that describe the pros and cons and the unknowns of using the medication. On the other hand, most people like to feel the material before they purchase the garment. Getting your own personal feel for a medication is a variation on that theme. But, if you do plan on continuing to use the medication, you must do something more objective than to take the detail man's word for its usefulness or to base its use on your own limited experience. To do otherwise does not live up to the standards of professional self-education, is not in the best interests of your patients, and it can cause harm to them.

In the practice of general pediatrics, the investment of the time and effort needed to learn about the new medications promoted by drug companies is not difficult; there are not many new ones. General pediatricians have a limited pharmacopeia, mainly antibiotics, infant formulas, antihistamines and decongestants, ointments and creams, analgesics and antipyretics, and anti-asthma medications.

It is essential to remember to remain your own and the patient's agent, rather than become the agent of the drug company that brings the gifts, no matter how inconsequential they seem. I believe, in the main, that this does happen. And I believe that, because of recent changes in the delivery of health care — more physicians practicing in groups, combined with the increased oversight (profiling) of physicians in order to hold down the costs of care — there will be a decreased ability of drug companies to influence the prescribing habits of physicians.

Pediatrician's Offices as a Pharmacy

The prescribing of medications by physicians is usual practice. The dispensing of medications by physicians is not, except under certain circumstances. As described above, the dispensing of samples to the patient at the point of contact for an illness is common practice. The patient receives a small amount of medication at no cost and presumably receives the rest at a pharmacy. The dispensing of medication by physicians as a profit-making enterprise is uncommon except in rural areas, where access to a pharmacy is difficult for the patient. In recent years, as physician fees have decreased and as drug prices have increased, the interest in dispensing drugs in physicians' offices has increased.[3,4,5]

An obvious conflict of interest exists when physicians dispense, for profit, medications which the patient can only obtain by a prescription from the physician. This conflict exists even when the medications are offered at prices that are lower than those available at outside pharmacies. The AAP has discussed this subject in both its committees on bioethics and on practice.[6,7,8,9,10,11] Without argument, the practice of charging the patient for medications dispensed in the office is an attempt by the physician to increase practice income. The fact that it may be less costly or more convenient, arguments that are used and are likely to be true, does not change the fact that it constitutes an inherent conflict of interest for the physician.

As with other ethical decisions, one must decide whether or not the other considerations overbalance the concerns raised by the conflict. Will the conflict of interest compromise the ability of the pediatrician to prescribe the most appropriate antibiotic, i.e., the one that is less profitable for the pediatrician but less expensive for the patient and just as effective? Will the lack of oversight by a pharmacist result in the use of a less effective medication, possibly resulting in a less favorable outcome for the patient? Will the profit motive result in *more* prescriptions being written? Will there be more errors in dispensing medications as a side-line in a busy office? Will the patient suffer from the lack of a second check by an independent pharmacist? These are difficult questions for an individual practitioner to answer and may, in fact, be the reason that the practice of establishing a pharmacy in the office has not become more widespread.

In the case of rural practices, where access for the patient to a commercial pharmacy is limited by distance, the use of the physician's office to provide pharmacy services appears, on balance, to be warranted. According to the AAP guidelines, however, if the physician wishes to provide a pharmacy service, he should charge what is reasonable, based on actual and overhead costs, and must also meet the safety standards seen in commercial pharmacies. These include keeping current with drug interactions and adverse effects, maintaining appropriate records, allowing refills without charging for office visits, and keeping stock current.

PEDIATRICIAN-PATIENT/FAMILY RELATIONSHIPS

At this point it is useful to establish a limited conceptual framework within which general pediatricians look at ethical issues. Pellegrino[12] states that much of recent bioethics is based on 4 general principles, as described by Beauchamp and Childress: nonmaleficence, beneficence, autonomy, and justice.[13] The first two, nonmaleficence and beneficence, correspond to the old Hippocratic principles of "do no harm" and "act in the best interests of the patient". Autonomy is a more recent principle. It deals with the right of the patient to have a major voice, if not *the* major voice, in health care decisions. It seems to have been embraced by the pediatricians interviewed, especially when dealing with mature adolescents. Justice, as a principle, when it deals with balancing the competing interests and claims of different family members does enter into the patient-physician relationship. When it deals with issues of fairness and access to care, the principle of justice enters into the private office chiefly as a question of how much uncompensated or under-compensated care a physician ought to provide. Experience gained from the interviews shows that the presence of a third party — the health insurer, whether governmental or private — exacerbates questions of fairness and access to care in the patient-pediatrician equation.

In the clinical examples that the practicing pediatricians discussed, there was strong evidence of their acceptance and use of the first three of these principles, despite their lack of formal exposure to these precepts. This is an important observation as it illustrates the incorporation into mainstream pediatrics of generally accepted ethical principles without exposure to formal learning.

The most vivid clinical examples came from stories of teenagers presenting with sexually transmitted diseases (STDs), pregnancy and drug use. The initial attitude when an adolescent presented with a need for confidentiality was that the adolescent had a right to have that need respected. The diagnosis was established and the appropriate treatment and counselling given. Whether the parents were informed was decided on a case by case basis.

Case One: A 17 year old female presented to the pediatrician with what proved to be genital warts. The teenager did not wish her parents to know the etiology of the infection. This request was respected. The pediatrician knew the girl and the family well and encouraged her to tell her parents about the etiology of her infection. She counselled her about telling her partner to be examined for sexually transmitted diseases, about pregnancy avoidance, the consequences of sexually transmitted diseases, especially with regard to human immunodeficiency virus (HIV) transmission, and the association of genital warts with papilloma virus infection and the potential for cervical cancer. This young woman was referred to a gynecologist with whom the pediatrician had consulted on similar cases in the past. The gynecologist's practice in these situations was to explain to parents that the medical history was confidential and would not be discussed with the parents unless the patient (the adolescent) requested it. The parents did not ask about the etiology of the infection, although the pediatrician believes that the parents did know. In this instance, the pediatrician and the gynecologist preserved the patients confidentiality because they trusted her autonomy, i.e., they did not tell the parents the cause of her infection, because of their assessment that she was mature enough to be treated as an adult. The pediatrician felt that it was in the patient's best interests (beneficence), and that no harm (nonmaleficence) would come from not telling.

***Comment*:** What criteria should be used by the pediatrician and the gynecologist to determine that someone is "mature enough" to be treated as an adult? Legal status is one factor; a 17 year old is pretty close to the legal definition of maturity. This should be coupled with other factors, such as the assessment of levels of emotional and intellectual development, as determined by past history and school performance, and an assessment of the present emotional state of the patient. If, after being encouraged to share the problem with her parents, the patient declines and offers reasonable arguments why her parents should not be told, a decision that she is "mature enough" can be made.

Case Two: A 15 year old pregnant female presented to the pediatrician early in the first trimester, requesting a referral for an abortion. She was a "young" 15 year old, was not in a long-term relation with a partner, and did not want her parents told about the pregnancy. The pediatrician confirmed the diagnosis and told the girl that she must tell her parents. The girl refused, stating that her parents would "kill her". The pediatrician did not accept this, stating that he did not believe her parents would "kill" her, and further stating that if the girl did not tell her parents the pediatrician would. Heeding the pediatrician's advice, the girl went home, told her parents, was not "killed", and had the abortion. In this instance, the pediatrician, who knew both the girl and the family well, made the assessment that respecting the patient's confidentiality was not in her best interest (beneficence) and might cause her harm (nonmaleficence).

***Comment*:** When does the pediatrician have the right (obligation) to override the child's decision to not tell her parents? What factors allow the pediatrician to determine that the patient's right to confidentiality should be overridden? The patient was 15 years old; that is sufficiently far from 18, the age of legal maturity, to use a high standard of proof in order to honor the request for confidentiality. The patient should demonstrate that a mature decision-making process has occurred. At a minimum, this should include thoughts about how to pay for the procedure and who was going to be her emotional support before, during, and after the procedure. If the reason for not informing her parents is fear of physical or emotional reprisals, some past evidence for this should be required. If the patient continues to have significant anxiety, the pediatrician should consider being with her when the parents are informed.

Case Three: A 17 year old pregnant female presented to the pediatrician requesting an abortion. She came with her partner, a young man with whom she had a long term relationship which they expected to continue. She did not want her parents told, explaining that they had recently gone through a great deal of family stress dealing with the prolonged illness of another family member. She did not believe that her parents would handle the news of her pregnancy well. She had, however, told her older sister with whom she had a close relationship. The sister agreed that the parents should not be told. The pediatrician agreed not to tell the parents and helped arrange for the abortion. The young woman had the support of her partner and her older sister at the time of the procedure. In this instance the pediatrician's assessment was that the patient should be treated as a mature adult, that the decision not to tell her parents was reasonable, and that the patient's confidentiality should be respected. The pediatrician believed that it was in the best interests (beneficence) of the young woman to do so and that no harm to the patient would be done by not telling (nonmaleficence).

***Comment*:** When should the pediatrician honor a patient's request for confidentiality? The answer to this question is embedded in the statements made in the previous cases. The patient should be judged to be mature, have made appropriate plans, and have demonstrated appropriate reasons for not telling the parents.

Case Four: The parents of a 15 year old boy asked their pediatrician to test their son's urine for drugs without informing the boy. The parent's reason for the request was that the boy's school performance had dropped off and his behavior had changed. He had become surly, and was away from home much of the time. The parents were known by the pediatrician to be concerned, sensitive individuals. On questioning by the pediatrician, the parents felt there was no evidence of severe depression in the child; they just believed that he was not "himself".

Despite some initial concern that he was not doing the "right thing", on a pretext, the pediatrician did obtain a urine sample from the boy, which did test positive for metabolites of marijuana. While awaiting the results of the urine test, the pediatrician had some concerns about the ethics of his testing for drug usage without informing the boy. He discussed the problem with his associates and the parents. It was agreed that the best course of action was for the pediatrician to confront the young man about the deterioration in his school performance and suggest that he, the pediatrician, was concerned that it might be related to drug use. He would not tell the boy that he had already tested his urine. When the confrontation took place the boy readily admitted to using marijuana on a daily basis, was concerned about what it was doing to him, and was eager to get some help. The boy was not told that his urine had been tested for drugs.

***Comment*:** Is it appropriate to test the urine for the presence of illicit drugs without first telling the patient? In this instance, the pediatrician felt that he had embarked on the wrong course, told the parents of his concern, readjusted, and confronted the child, who admitted to illicit drug use.

Covert drug testing is a poor substitute for developing open communications and voluntary cooperation. On reflection, both the parents and the pediatrician agreed that the initial course of action should have been to confront the boy about the possibility of drug use as the cause of his behavioral changes. If he had denied the use of drugs they could have asked him to produce a urine sample at that time, explaining that it would be tested for drugs. In terms of practical benefits and harms, there was time to act in a less precipitous fashion, since his life was not thought to be in danger. Having the boy involved in the decision-making process was more likely to be successful in the long term. Trust is difficult to re-establish once it has been betrayed. However, had the child appeared to have been severely depressed, and had there been concern about the possibility of suicide, then beneficence might justifiably overrule respect for autonomy.

The major principle in this case is respect for the patient's autonomy. For autonomy to be abridged there needs to be some overriding reason, such as evidence of self-destructive behavior. This view is consistent with the AAP's guidelines on the screening for drugs of abuse.[14] In the above case this condition did not appear to have been met. The decision, therefore, whether or not to respect the autonomy of the adolescent should be based on principles similar to those of the first three cases described.

The principle of autonomy was also of concern in another type of clinical situation. A few pediatricians were trying to answer the question whether or not families should participate in the decision making process when the current weight of medical opinion did not support routine use of a particular treatment. The problem was especially interesting if the family had no knowledge of the therapy, requiring the pediatrician to raise the question if they were to be able to make a choice.

Several clinical examples were given. The first was the use of oral acyclovir to mitigate the severity of chicken pox in normal children. The current recommendation by the American Academy of Pediatrics is to reserve the routine use of oral acyclovir in a patient with chicken pox to those children with a co-existing immune problem, such as children with human immunodeficiency virus (HIV) infection, or for children who have been treated for acute leukemia.[15]*

Uncompromised children who received acyclovir were able to return to school about one day earlier than children who had not.[16] For some parents, that one day might be important, especially if both parents worked and had problems with day care when their children were ill. The arguments against using acyclovir are simple: while the drug is generally judged to be safe, it is an anti-metabolite and the long term effects of its use in young children are unknown. (Remember, the adverse effects of diethyl stilbesterol (DES) were not known until many years after its initial use.) In addition, using a medication for a self-limited illness for minimal benefit is costly, since almost every child will develop chicken pox.

Other examples were: the use of amantadine to decrease the severity of, or for prophylaxis of, influenza A; the use of Hemophilus influenzae B vaccine in children older than 5 years of age; and the use of Hepatitis B vaccine in children who were not newborns or teenagers. In all of these examples, certain children who might benefit from these treatments fall outside the official recommendations. Should pediatricians discuss these issues with their families, allowing them to decide on a case by case basis whether they wish

*Author's note: Since writing this article, varicella vaccination has been approved for routine use in the U.S. It is reasonable to assume that acyclovir issue may become moot, but the illustration is still valid.

their children to receive the treatment? In other words, should the consideration of *parent* autonomy to make close-call decisions be respected? It is always most difficult to respect parents' autonomy when we disagree with their choices. If their choices are clearly harmful they must be opposed. The difficult issues arise when the risks to the child of agreeing are small, and the injury to the parents of refusing are great.

When the pediatrician who initially posed the problem was asked how he became concerned with these borderline issues, he explained that many years ago he had seen a two year old who had become deaf in one ear following a bout of mumps. He had been tempted to immunize all his patients. But at that time mumps vaccine had just been developed and was only being recommended for adolescent males, to avoid mumps-associated orchitis. Subsequently, as more vaccine became available and more experience with the vaccine was gained, the recommendations were changed to include all children.

All good practitioners know they must be careful using the "Burn Method" of learning, i.e., once burned, always learned, one individual experience should not be generalized to apply to all patients. But, good practitioners also know that flexibility and adaptability are necessary in order to be responsible to new information and open to improved procedures.

***Summary*:** The stories the pediatricians told demonstrated a high level of thoughtfulness in decision-making around ethical issues. This developed not from formal training in the field of bioethics but rather from the need to find rational and practical solutions to difficult clinical situations. Pediatricians who practice primary care have the welfare of their patients as their primary clinical concern. Therefore, it is not surprising that they would wish to act in the patient's best interests and to do no harm. It is surprising that the principle of autonomy is given such respect, even among the pediatricians trained in the 1960's, when the central role of the patient in the decision-making process was not well-developed. Nevertheless, they are beginning to require evidence of potential harm to the patient before they are willing to abridge the right to autonomy. I believe this to be an appropriate shift, consistent with current developments in bioethics and with societal and patient expectations.

PEDIATRICIAN-HEALTH INSURER RELATIONSHIPS

Great passion, which often bordered on great anger, was aroused when the pediatricians interviewed were asked questions about how health insurers affected their practice of medicine. The conversation would usually begin by a discussion about how much fun pediatric practice had been in the past and how little fun it was now. The reason identified for the decrease in the joy of practice was the intrusion of health insurers. In many parts of the country, it was not until the 1980's that "Managed Care" took hold. In 1973, 5 million people were enrolled in health maintenance organizations (HMOs); by 1991 this had increased to 36 million.[17] The effect on the fee-for-service general pediatrician was to introduce insurance forms, pre-authorization for certain tests and procedures, and loss of patients when a change in health insurance no longer covered their services.

The pediatricians' passion was focused on their perception that, somehow or other, the limitations placed on them by insurance company requirements had decreased the quality of the care their patients received. In fact, there is support for this position in the recent literature.[18] The argument put forward is that limiting the physician's ability to act in the best interests of the patient will, *a fortiuri*, force decisions to be made that adversely affect outcome. These physicians frame their arguments in terms of the ethical principle of justice. Justice relates to fairness. It is unfair, the pediatricians believe, to limit or restrict benefits just because the health insurer wants to save money. Ironically, had they done what the health insurer wanted, it would have cost the insurer more money in some instances. The argument could also be made that the operative ethical principle is autonomy-that patients and their families have a right to unrestricted choice of beneficial care. However, unrestricted patient or doctor choice does not always produce improved outcomes in health status.

Case One: A 12 year old girl presented to the pediatrician with a 7 week history of diarrhea. The child had been well until about 2 months prior to this episode when she developed an abcess in her ear lobe due to an earring. In addition to local treatment, she was given an antibiotic. The infection cleared, but she developed diarrhea. A work-up for the possibility of Clostridium difficile-associated diarrhea was negative.

The father had a past history of lactose intolerance versus celiac disease. The pediatrician felt it would be easier to rule in or out the diagnosis of lactose intolerance, and that the most accurate noninvasive test he knew was a breath hydrogen determination. Before ordering the test he needed to get pre-authorization from the health insurer. But, he got someone on the line who told him that a breath hydrogen test was not on their list of approved tests. He then asked to speak to the medical director, who was unavailable. A day or so later someone else called him up to tell him that the medical director had not heard of a breath hydrogen test and therefore would not approve it. At this point, the pediatrician could have given up and asked for a consultation with a pediatric gastroenterologist. This would have cost the health insurer more, and introduced the patient to another physician who might possibly have ordered more expensive and more invasive tests. Instead, he persisted, finally reached the medical director, explained his reasoning, and got the test approved.

Case Two: An 8 year old boy was brought to the pediatrician's office complaining of pain in his ankle following a fall while playing soccer. The ankle was swollen with some point tenderness, but there was no deformity. The pediatrician could not rule out the possibility of a non-displaced fracture and wanted to obtain a radiograph of the ankle. The parents belonged to a health insurance plan that required the use of a particular local radiology group. The pediatrician called that group, but no one was available to interpret the film until the next day. There was another radiology group nearby, and they did have someone available to take and interpret the radiograph immediately. However, this group was not on the list approved by the patient's health insurer. The nearest approved radiologist who could take and interpret the film immediately was *20 miles away.*

These facts were explained to the health insurer's representative on the telephone by the pediatrician. Using the non-approved nearby radiologist was not an option. The patient could go either to the office 20 miles away or to the local hospital emergency room.

The family was given the options by the pediatrician, and chose to go to the hospital emergency room. After waiting for over an hour, the radiograph was taken and interpreted as not showing any evidence of fracture by the emergency room physician. However, the emergency room physician was uncomfortable interpreting an ankle radiograph of an

8 year old, no radiologist was present in the hospital by this time, and an orthopedist was asked to see the child. The emergency room physician's interpretation was confirmed, a support bandage applied, and the child sent home to recuperate.

Case Three: A 4 year old boy had reconstructive cardiac surgery at 1 year of age for a major, complex cardiac malformation. He had now developed evidence of obstructive apnea related to enlarged adenoids and tonsils. He received his primary care from a pediatrician in the town in which he lived, and his health insurance was through a managed care plan. In conjunction with an otolaryngologist consultant, he decided to refer the child to the nearby academic center where the initial cardiac surgery was performed and where the child was still followed by a pediatric cardiologist.

Both consultants agreed that the child needed to have his adenoids and tonsils removed. The doctors wished to have the procedure done at the medical center where a pediatric anesthesiologist was available, as was a pediatric intensive care unit for post-operative observation. However, the health plan wanted the procedure done in the local hospital at which they received a discounted rate.

The pediatrician had to enter into prolonged negotiations with the health plan's medical director, who was not a pediatrician. He did not appreciate the known complications, including sudden respiratory arrest, that might arise post-operatively in this child and that required overnight observation in a pediatric intensive care unit. The pediatrician argued that if the health plan insisted on the child being operated on at the local hospital then they had to accept the medical liability. After more discussion and more forms to be filled out, the health plan agreed to allow the operation to be done at the medical center.

***Comment*:** These three cases are illustrative of many others the author heard. All of them have the same plot; a knowledgeable and concerned pediatrician wants to care for the patient using either the least intrusive and most economical diagnostic and treatment plan, or the most appropriate management plan even though the initial cost might be higher. Obstacles are placed in the way by the health insurer, obstacles that are not designed to improve the care of the patient, but to decrease the cost of care. And, in many of these scenarios, the care actually rendered turns out to be not only less beneficial, but also more costly.

The principles of beneficence and justice are applicable in these cases. The pediatricians believed that they and their patients were being dealt with unjustly and that decisions they were asked to make by health insurers were based on reducing the cost of health care, with little or no regard for the quality of the care delivered. It seems apparent that a divergence of interests exists between corporate providers of care and individual receivers of care. At times, that conflict poses real risks that doing what is in the patient's best interests will be compromised.

SUMMARY

In this chapter I have tried to determine the major ethical issues in the private practice of general pediatrics, using as my vantage point the experiences and practices of individual pediatricians. I sought out pediatricians whose views I believed to be in the mainstream of the best and most thoughtful clinicians. It was a biased sample, and the chapter reflects my own biases also. Viewing how health care is delivered in this way is different than the prism through which academic ethicists' generally look at issues; it is a bottom up, rather than a top-down, approach. Why should the opinions of these unnamed and unnumbered individuals be regarded as authoritative, as normative for others? Is the authority here more than merely anecdotal? Despite the limited and biased sample, I believe the answer to both these questions is "Yes!" Pediatricians see patients one by one, case by case. The decisions they make grow out of years and years of weighing the details of individual cases. Their judgements have been refined and proven by the ultimate test: the effect on thousands of real patients and their families. The principles of their practice have been proven *in* their practice.

References

1. Editorial, Gifts to Physicians from Industry, Council on Ethics and Judicial Affairs of American Medical Association, *JAMA,* **265**, p. 501.
2. Getting good value from drug reps. (1983). *Drug Ther. Bull.,* **21**:13–15.
3. Margolis, L. H., (1991). The ethics of accepting gifts from pharmaceutical companies. *Pediatrics,* **88**:1233–1237.
4. Statement on Office-Based Medication dispensing in Pediatric Practice, Committee on Practice and Ambulatory Medicine, American Academy of Pediatrics. *Pediatrics,* **83**:143–144.
5. Letter to American Academy of Pediatrics, Dyer, Ellis, Joseph and Mills (law firm), April, 1987.
6. Prescription-Drug Sale by Doctors is Opposed. The New York Times, March 22, 1987.
7. Number of Doctors Selling Prescription Drugs Grows, The New York Times, March 19, 1987.
8. Statement of Policy Regarding Relationships With Pharmaceutical Companies. (AAP) Draft, March 18, 1985.
9. Memorandum, Office Dispensing of Drugs, April 7, (1987). American Academy of Pediatrics.
10. Office Dispensing of Drugs, Draft Statement, Practice Committee, American Academy of Pediatrics. February 18, 1988.
11. Hoopes, J. M. Letter to Doctors from Physicians' Pharmaceutical Services, Inc., September 8, 1987.
12. Pellegrino, E. D. (1993). The Metamorphosis of Medical Ethics, A 30-year Perspective. *JAMA,* **269**:1158–1162.
13. Beauchamp, T. L., Childress, J. F., *Principles of Biomedical Ethics.* Oxford University Press, New York, Oxford 1979.
14. Screening for Drugs of Abuse in Children and Adolescents, Statement by Committee on Adolescence, Committee on Bioethics, and Provisional Committee on Substance Abuse, American Academy of Pediatrics (1989). *Pediatrics,* **84**:396–397.
15. Varicella-Zoster (1991). Infections, Report of the Committee on Infectious Diseases, American Academy of Pediatrics.
16. Balfour, H. H., Jr., Kelly, J. M., Suarez, C. S., *et al.*, (1990). Acyclovir Treatment of Varicella in Otherwise Healthy Children. *J. Pediatr.,* **116**:633–639.
17. MacLeod G. K. (1993) An overview of managed health care. In: *The Managed Health Care Handbook* edited by Kongstvedt, P. R. 2nd Edition, Aspen: Gaithersburg, MD.
18. Emanuel, E. J. and Brett, A. S. (1993). Managed competition and the patient-physician relationship, sounding board. *New England Journal of Medicine,* **329**:879–882.

8 All in the Family: The Inequity Between Parental Rights and Home Care Duties

Alex Okun

Albert Einstein College of Medicine, Bronx Municipal Hospital Center, Pelham Parkway South and Eastchester Road, Bronx, New York 10461, USA

Almost everyone has provided home care to another person at some time. Many children have grown up helping care for sick siblings, parents or elderly relatives. Those who have never nursed a sick family member have probably had to perform duties neglected by others who did.

Parents' duties in home care are extensions of their everyday obligations to provide food and shelter, education, medical care and a stable family for their children. As families have taken sicker children home from the hospital, the limits of their home care obligations have been stretched to the extreme.[1] However, existing rights and the choices available to parents are insufficient to enable many to fulfill these duties. The consequences of this inequity are borne entirely by the child and family.

In this chapter, I will focus on the rights and choices parents have been granted and the increasing duties expected of them in home care today. I will illustrate the inequity between parental rights and duties with the stories of three families with whom I have worked in home care. I will suggest some ways the medical community and society at large can help shrink this gap by reassessing its expectations of parents and bolstering their rights and freedom to make decisions in home care.

FOOD AND SHELTER: THE CASE OF DEREK

Derek was born after placental abruption at 25 weeks' gestation to a 32-year-old registered nurse, a mother of three. He weighed 570 grams at birth and received aggressive resuscitative treatment for close to 1 hour. He remained ventilator-dependent for several months and eventually required a tracheostomy to bypass tracheal narrowing caused by the mechanical ventilation. He was severely brain-damaged and fed poorly.

The mother visited nightly. She quickly learned to care for the tracheostomy. On the medical floor where she worked in the same hospital, she was known as one of the best staff nurses at techniques such as ostomy care and tube placement. She was able to feed Derek larger volumes of formula than most of the pediatric nursing staff could.

When Derek was first born, his mother did not think he would survive. She grew strongly attached to him over the first months and could not consider separating from him on a long-term basis. When he was medically stable, a 1 or 2 month placement in a pediatric rehabilitation facility was offered as an alternative to taking him home. The usual goal of this sort of placement is to help a caregiver master the skills necessary to take the child home. Derek's mother was proficient at these procedures before he was born. She was not offered a more long-term placement alternative, as the staff were sure that she was able and wanted to care for him at home.

Derek's mother was encouraged by the staff's confidence in her and agreed that taking him home was the best decision for everyone involved. She thought that her family could ensure his developmental progress better than the staff in an institution. She spent long hours visiting Derek in the hospital and saw his discharge as a way to be around home more with her three other children. Derek was sent home at 6 months of age on continuous oxygen, frequent suctioning, oral feedings and nebulized medication treatments, with home nursing services in place 14 hours a day.

The next 6 months were trying. Derek had three laser treatments to remove tracheal scar tissue, with little improvement. He gained weight poorly and developed urinary tract infections. Tube feedings were started to help him grow. By 1 year of age, he was able to smile responsively and follow objects to some extent. Tests revealed that he was profoundly deaf.

Variations in the mother's monthly earnings resulted in her Medicaid and Social Security Disability benefits being alternatively cut off and reinstated. She had to take unscheduled days off from work when Derek's home nurse arrived late or a substitute was sent. She accrued no vacation time. Her toddler daughter demanded more attention, and her 8- and 11-year-old boys began to have problems in school. Derek's father lived outside the home, visited erratically and remained uninvolved with him. Derek's mother became pregnant by the father and needed an emergency operation for an ectopic pregnancy.

At the end of the year, Derek's mother regretted the decision she had made to take Derek home. She felt that she had made her choice from limited alternatives, and ignorant of whether it would truly serve the best interests of Derek or the others in her family. As she looked back over the first 6 months at home, she saw little developmental or physical progress and felt that her personal and family life were falling apart. She foresaw future procedures of uncertain efficacy and worried that Derek would suffer needlessly. She questioned whether it had all been worth it.

It is only in the past decade that children like Derek had any hope of surviving the neonatal period. Twenty years ago, it was considered unusual to expect parents to be able to care at home for infants with tracheostomies,[2] or those on continuous oxygen.[3] An otherwise healthy child with Derek's mental and motor impairments would most likely have been placed in an institution.

As the public learned more about the impact of maternal deprivation and impersonal treatment on the development of children in such institutions,[4] families began being asked to consider taking their mentally impaired children home to live. Most physicians still recommended institutional placement to the parents of children with Down's Syndrome born in the 1940's and 50's. Several groups of such parents were the subjects of reports from Denmark,[5] Scotland[6] and the United States.[7] In the beginning, these parents felt they could not live without their infants and believed it was best for them to be home. Families who later institutionalized their children did so due to exhaustion, departure of one or both parents, disturbance to other family members, or the sense that it had become "best for the child".

Over the next half century, the medical establishment and society in general strengthened in their conviction that home was "best" for children like Derek. Enthusiasm about home care shifted from families with mentally impaired children to those whose children had complex medical needs. As the care of sick newborns became more effective, families were asked to take home fragile infants who previously would not have been expected to live. One group of parents of neonatal intensive care unit survivors from the 1960's and 1970's feared that in choosing to care for their infants at home, "they and their other children would become socially enslaved, economically deprived and permanently stigmatized, all perhaps for a lost cause".[8]

Recently, the virtues of taking home children who are extremely medically complex or dependent on technology have been extolled. The home has been hailed as a "safe environment for all",[9] full of "opportunities for spiritual growth and wellness",[10] where appropriate education, developmental interaction and stimulation from friends can occur. The home has been credited with "normalizing the lives" of some children dependent on technology,[11] and with enabling families to grow closer and helping siblings become more sensitive adults.[12] Compared to the dark images of children in institutions, home care has come to be viewed as "a paradigm of choice"[13] and in the best interests of children with chronic illness and their families.[14]

Derek's mother feels that she did not have much of a choice whether to accept or reject this paradigm. However, she has found none of the "virtues" of home care to be the reality for her family. The sorts of problems she has confronted in home care have not been emphasized in reports of successful home care programs for children with chronic illness. Many studies of technology-dependent children living at home have included descriptions of such "complications",[15] but none have been able to distinguish the burdens of chronic illness from the effects of caring for a child with chronic illness at home.

Few long-term alternatives to home care exist for children like Derek that are acceptable to parents and medical staff. Derek's doctors and nurses offered none. This deficit leaves many parents with little choice but to try their best, against great odds, to provide food and shelter at home.

In the last section of this chapter, I will offer suggestions for ways the in-patient medical team and family can best look at whether home care plans are likely to succeed, or even ought to be considered in the first place. In the next section, I will explore another area in which parents feel they have gained little autonomy in spite of great legislative advances over the past 20 years.

EDUCATION: THE CASE OF DENNIS

Dennis was a 14-year-old boy who qualified for special education services because of moderate mental retardation, hearing impairment and club foot. He also had asthma, a tracheostomy, pituitary insufficiency, chronic mastoiditis and behavior problems.

When Dennis was 12 years old, his foot was put in a cast after a surgical procedure performed before the start of summer school. He was not able to walk easily with crutches, and his mother asked for physical therapy services from the school. The school did not offer these services. It sent her a list of clinics that accepted Medicaid and asked that she use one of these.

Dennis' mother found it burdensome to transport him for treatment in the community and argued that he should be entitled to care in his school. The school administrator defended its position, as she had not forewarned the school of Dennis' elective surgery or given it time to anticipate his needs in the midst of a lightly staffed summer session.

Dennis' foot began to hurt. His mother did not respond to letters from the school urging her to seek medical attention for his pain. As she saw it, the pain was caused by the school's failure to provide him the physical therapy to which she thought he was entitled. The school reported her to child protective services for medical neglect. By the time the investigation was underway, the cast had been removed, the pain had abated and an orthopedist declared that Dennis could walk well enough so that he did not need physical therapy any more.

Dennis' mother never complained formally to the school about its failure to provide physical therapy. The report to child protective services infuriated her. She withdrew him from school, believing she could teach him more at home than the school could. She asked his doctors, "How can he learn to read and write or become independent in a class full of wild retarded boys?"

Rather than appeal against those aspects of the educational plan which she felt to be inadequate or too restrictive, Dennis' mother obtained certification to teach him at home. His medical providers told her that while they suspected she was probably qualified to teach him the material, withdrawing him from the social milieu of school was not in his best interests. To them, her solution seemed to be at odds with her desire to help Dennis achieve greater independence. Having tried to avoid shuttling Dennis to and from physical therapy, she ended up with a commitment to spend many more hours a day teaching him at home.

Parents have the moral obligation to see that their children learn as much about the world as they can and grow into independent, effective, feeling adults. They hope their children will develop meaningful commitments to rewarding work and enriching relationships with others.

The reality of these aspirations is challenged by the disabilities of many children who require specialized home care. Those with mental handicaps may never be able to live independently. Others surviving with physical disorders may be limited in the scope of their work potential and hindered in their relations with friends and family. Legislation enacted in the 1970's and 1980's in the United States created educational opportunities for children like Dennis and standardized methods for parents to take advantage of them. All professionals working with children should be knowledgeable about these laws.

The provisions set out in Public Law 94-142, the "Education for All Handicapped Children Act of 1975", did more to advance the educational rights and opportunities of children who receive some form of home care than any other piece of legislation.[16] This law established a set of minimum requirements that special education programs must meet in order for states to receive certain federal funds. Special education and "related services" must be individually designed to meet the needs of eligible children and be provided year-round in "the least restrictive environment".

The law pertains to children defined as handicapped with defects such as mental retardation, specific learning disability, hearing or speech impairment, visual handicap, serious emotional disturbance or other multiple handicaps. "Related services" are mandated for children with handicaps to help eliminate potential barriers to education. Examples of related services include transportation, speech pathology, audiology, physical and occupation therapy, recreation, diagnostic evaluation, school health services, psychological testing and counselling, social work and parent training and counselling.

PL 94-142 applies to children aged 5 to 21 years. Public Law 99-457, the "Education of the Handicapped Act Amendments of 1986", extends these rights to children with disabilities aged 3 to 5 years. Qualified state programs also provide evaluative services and intervention to infants from birth to age 3 years who have been determined to be at risk of developmental disability. PL 99-457 requires that services be provided for the family as a whole.[17] Written plans must address the needs of parents and siblings as well as the child targeted for intervention.

While many children receiving some form of home care are eligible for special education and related services under these laws, some children with chronic illness do not meet criteria which would classify them as needing special education or being developmentally at risk. It is unclear to what extent support services should be provided for those children who require related services but can function in a regular classroom[18] — for example, a school-age child with normal intelligence needing physical therapy for mild leg spasticity. Even when children do qualify for special education, the gap between their needs and available resources may be wide. A study of related services provided in 1983 to children with special needs in five large metropolitan areas revealed that a sizable minority enrolled in special education were not receiving services specific to their disability.[19]

Parents may object to any part of the special educational plan offered for their child informally or in writing. This complaint initiates the appeals process, which starts with an "impartial due process hearing". The results of this hearing can be appealed to the level of the state education agency, and beyond there to state or federal courts. The agency ultimately responsible for related services is not the school district or the medical establishment, but the educational agency of the state.[20] The family's distance from this bureaucratic locus of responsibility makes it even less clear for parents where to turn to demand related services for their children. The complaint, hearing and appeals process is expensive, complicated and beyond the reach of many families. Many parents cannot tolerate any better than Dennis' mother some of the steps they must take to advocate for their children's right to special education and related services. Even the most sophisticated and litigious parents become exhausted and alienated in the process.

Parents must check their hopes and dreams for their children's futures against the realistic limits on their capacity to make these dreams come true. The parents of one handicapped child wrote that they balanced urges to become the "best damn parents" with the need to be more self-centered.[21] The best long-term approach to education for them, and for Dennis' mother, lies somewhere between complacency and tireless advocacy.

Parental adequacy and authority are challenged in dealings with the in-patient medical and special education bureaucracies. In the next section, I will describe some of the ways coordinating out-patient medical treatment can be just as difficult for families involved in home care.

MEDICAL CARE: THE CASE OF DARLENE

Darlene was a healthy, overweight 19-month-old girl who developed a severe systemic herpes virus infection and was hospitalized with encephalitis and respiratory failure. This resulted in a seizure disorder, mild mental retardation, motor deficits and chronic lung disease. She required 4 months of mechanical ventilation in intensive care and was transferred to the "respirator unit" of a pediatric rehabilitation facility for 1 year. By her third birthday, Darlene was discharged home on a respirator around the clock, with nursing services in place 24 hours a day.

The 45-year-old father suffered from diabetes, heart and peptic ulcer disease and was heavily dependent on the 30-year-old mother. She complained that he did not take responsibility for Darlene's care, even when a nurse was in the home. Darlene soon went off to preschool with her respirator and other equipment packed into a little red wagon, pulled behind her by her nurse. After 9 months, nursing services were no longer needed overnight.

Darlene's obesity worsened in the first year home. Her mother became enraged whenever the primary care team urged attention to the weight problem. She blamed the obesity on steroid medication given a year earlier and accused the team of racist insensitivity to her family's "genetic disposition to big bones". The team learned from nurses in the home that Darlene's father fed her pints of ice cream at a sitting and that her mother provided her other high-calorie snacks.

Darlene's mother sought to obtain an exercise bicycle through Medicaid to enable her daughter to "work off the weight". The team counseled her that it was not a developmentally appropriate method of weight control and did not assist her in applying for the bicycle. A short time later, she asked for a potty seat made specifically for large children, also through Medicaid. She had chosen this item, listed at a price of several hundred dollars, from a vendor's catalogue. A standard bedside commode "would not do," according to the mother. When the primary care team declined to assist her in this request, the mother sought approval, in turn, from the neurologist, pulmonologist, developmental pediatrician and psyciatrist involved in Darlene's care. On a home visit a short time later, the team discovered the new exercise bicycle and special potty seat in the living room.

The mother attempted to wean Darlene from the respirator in ways that led to frequent disputes with the medical staff. "I leave her off it at home", she would say. "She knows when she needs the machine — she comes running back for it!" Darlene's parents believed that her developing lungs would not grow unless challenged. The pulmonologist and primary care team thought her lungs should be supported while they grew and worried that undertreatment might hasten the development of circulatory problems related to the lung disease.

By the time Darlene was 5 years old, the pulmonologist and primary care team agreed that she had improved enough that she needed the ventilator only when she slept. While awake, she could move about safely on continuous oxygen, off the machine. Nurses reported that Darlene spent much of her time at home off oxygen altogether, against medical advice. Several nurses left or were fired by the family over this conflict.

Darlene enrolled in kindergarten on continuous oxygen. A year later, her mother asked for it to be discontinued. She said she wanted Darlene to be able to play more freely with her friends, rather than remain "tethered to the oxygen like an animal on a leash". After several meetings, the primary care team, mother and home nurse together devised a plan to monitor Darlene's oxygen saturation and clinical signs off oxygen for a 3-week period.

Darlene desaturated quickly during this three-week trial, without showing clear physical signs of low oxygen. The entire group, including the mother, agreed that Darlene could not be weaned as yet. Her mother continued to leave her off oxygen much of the time at home but did not fight to remove the oxygen at school as fervently as she had pursued equipment purchases in the past.

Dealing with the medical establishment is one of the most difficult duties for parents in home care. Darlene and her mother use an out-patient program for medical care that works better than most, providing home visits, easy accessibility and frequent communication with subspecialists and community services. Hospital out-patient clinics and private offices are usually organized to meet the needs of medical providers, subspecialists and finance departments, rather than families. "A clinic card, easily left home by mistake, can make the difference between rapid attention to a child and long hours of waiting."[22]

Children with a chronic illness or disability must often obtain their care at hospitals, which they depend on for admissions, special procedures and specialty care. Unlike Darlene's home care program, the organizational nature of most institutions provides little forum for communication between medical professionals.[23] Parents of chronically ill children may be forced to serve as the "case manager" for their child, attempting to correlate and communicate the views of many professionals. Parents are often ill-equiped to present the fine points of one doctor's thinking to another or to each other. Discussing medical decisions with the provider is a foreign concept to many parents from cultures in which great authority is vested in the doctor.[24] Some must struggle to raise their own literacy level or learn enough English and medical terminology to get by in the medical world.[25]

When questions about the child arise at home, parents may not know to whom to turn. Many specialists are elusive or unavailable, and many primary care practitioners are tentative and less well informed.[26] Parents must learn to individualize their communicative approach to different health professionals. They need to be more inquisitive and advocating with some, and more passive and deferential to others, lest they be viewed as "difficult".[27]

In spite of these tensions, parents are expected to trust the providers, believing that they have their child's and family's best interests at heart.[28] Darlene's mother has not been able fully to trust the medical establishment that "allowed" her child to become ill in the first place. Likewise, the team has not taken seriously some of her demands. As she begins to negotiate more effectively with the professional team, it will be able to work more patiently and collaboratively with her. It is their mutual obligation to learn to plan the home care of the child/patient together. In the next section, I will describe some of the effects of home care on the family that strain this effort at collaboration.

KEEPING THE FAMILY TOGETHER

The child with chronic illness or disability cannot be raised with food, shelter, education and medical care alone. The child needs "people to love [and] receive affection from ...

patterns for identification provided by the parents ... to be accepted, valued and wanted as a member of the family unit."[29] These ideals cannot always be achieved by families with children in home care. Parents like Derek's, Dennis' and Darlene's often feel guilty for failing to meet these needs and bitter at the expectation that they should be able to.

The demand to incorporate a "defective" child into the family system may threaten its very rules and boundaries.[30] The initial response of a family to the diagnosis of a child's chronic illness has been described as a mixture of fear, anxiety, anger, depression and guilt.[31] Many of these early feelings are reactivated as the child enters new developmental stages and whenever the disease flares.[32]

A state of "chronic sorrow"[33] can evolve in some families as the strains of time and financial commitment, modification of family activities, loss of privacy and social isolation intensify.[34] Cyclical states of terror, resentment, exhaustion, oppression and guilt[35] lead many parents to feel they have lost total control over their lives.[36] In order to salvage the family, some are urged to enter psychotherapy as individuals or a family unit, an engagement that would otherwise be completely foreign to them.

From an economic point of view, home care for children who are dependent on technology is far less costly than hospital care, except when the need for nursing services approaches 24 hours per day.[37] The principle source of cost savings comes from the substitution of parental services for professional nursing in the home. No one has yet been able to quantify the "opportunity costs" of home care: the price families pay due to lost opportunities to work, advance their careers or even shop more thriftily. Parents are ultimately liable for the expense of services received in the home, whether or not they have medical insurance. They must stand guard against "exploitative entrepreneurialism",[38] home care agencies which place services in the home for profit rather than for the patient's needs.

Beyond its emotional and financial threat to family integrity, chronic childhood illness is ultimately an affliction of the main parental caretaker, the mother. An unsupportive or absent father can be detrimental to the mother's acceptance of the child into the family from the infant's first days.[39] When the mother bears principal or sole responsibility for the child, she must consider how to care for the child and simultaneously tend to her own needs and those of the family, marriage or partnership.[40] She must learn new skills as a medical manager, financial planner, educational advocate, resource specialist and employer.[41] This sort of transformation is beyond the abilities of many.

A mother must learn to inflict pain as she masters procedures such as suctioning, tube placement and injections. This shift from her role as the protector and consoler of her child can obscure the boundaries of the traditional, comfort-based relationship between her and her child[42] and threaten the integrity of that relationship.

A mother, a parent, must do all this for the child. The medical team need not. Health care providers overwhelmed by the care of a child with complex medical needs may refer the child to another provider, program or hospital. Parents who discover that home care is "more than they signed up for" are not as free to choose among alternatives. Thus, the medical team is afforded a choice that parents are not: the choice to withdraw from the care of the child. Parents are expected never to retreat from their vigilant, compliant position in home care, lest they risk being labelled "neglectful", "uninvolved" or "difficult".

In the last section of this chapter, I will suggest ways the medical establishment and society in general can be less "neglectful" of, "uninvolved" with or "difficult" for the families of children with complex medical needs. By modifying the way decisions are made with families and encouraging them to fight for all the services they are entitled to, the medical establishment and society as a whole can augment parental rights and restore their freedom to choose in home care.

SUGGESTIONS

Changes in Hospital Policy

Therapeutic decisions during in-patient pediatrics are based mainly upon what hospital staff perceive to be the "best interests" of the child.[43] As shown during the Baby Doe years, society has come to assume that these interests are served best by going to great lengths to preserve the life of almost any child. Feinberg has written that decisions based on these assumptions can lead to "dependence on technology over quality of life concerns".[44]

Except for specific procedures requiring informed consent, the entire process of in-patient therapeutic decision-making in pediatrics often occurs without input from the family. Parents whose children survive intensive care admissions tethered to machines or dependent on numerous medications or procedures are often included for the first time in this process when they are informed that discharge is imminent.[45] Unaccustomed to autonomy in their child's care, many parents agree to take their child home without fully considering or being offered the alternatives. In so doing, many overestimate their own psychological competence to handle this terrifying challenge. Facing severe bed shortages in units filled with acutely and more critically ill children, in-patient staff are often as eager as the parents to believe that specific home care plans will work out well.

Most pediatric units have not developed standard methods to help parents make decisions about the commitment to care for a child with complex medical needs at home. Parents are assumed to prefer home care. They are shown what they need to know to survive the first few days at home and sent on their way with a list of phone numbers, a few shopping bags filled with supplies and equipment, and their child.

A family's moral duty to its critically ill members, even its children, must have limits.[46] John Hardwig asserts that it is the medical team's duty to consider the limits to which the mother and family can be asked to go. When it does not, the consequences for the child and family may be dire.[47]

In the process of deciding whether home care is appropriate to initiate or continue for a child, John Lantos and Arthur Kohrman have called for the construction of a "calculus of collective best interests" by which the benefits to the child and family are weighed against the burdens of care for other family members. Ideally, this calculus should be defined by the family, uninfluenced by the special interests of medical staff, hospital administrators or insurance companies.[48]

They have proposed several preconditions to home care. Before a home care plan is defined, parents must be willing to care for the child at home and know that providing such care is an extraordinary challenge. Medical staff must assure that the resources necessary for successful discharge will continue to be there in the future and take responsibility for the care of and advocacy for the child and family once they are home. Together, staff and family must define and agree on the goals of home care. In the authors' words, medical staff must take "responsibility" for these duties and remain "responsive" to family's needs.[49]

As the medical team enters into this process of "education and negotiation", it must initiate regular meetings with the family at the outset of hospitalization, not wait till discharge is planned. In some situations, medical staff may need to go to the family's home to meet key family members who cannot or will not come to the hospital at convenient times.

The medical team should consider involving an unbiased advisor who can help articulate the patient's, family's, medical staff's and hospital's interests. This could be a member of the clergy, mental health profession or institutional ethics committee. By helping explain each party's point of view to the others, such an advisor can defend against misunderstandings in the decision-making process. Coerced or uninformed choices to take ill children home have been termed, "doomed to failure, conflict and psychological discomfort".[50]

The family's decision to take home its ill child must stand the test of time. Excitement and interest in the child and family often subside as the crisis of discharge passes and the inevitable problems in home care emerge. Family members and friends who may have appeared to be sources of great potential support fade into the woodwork. Patterns of behavior which define the family's pattern of coping with their child's home care become clearer.

When home care is being considered from the in-patient unit, the primary care team that will handle the future medical care of the child must be involved early on. This team is more accustomed to sharing authority with parents in decision-making for their children. Once the child has been discharged, it can be responsive to subtle cues from family members asking for respite from home care. The team may recognize potential sources of help unapparent to the family in the midst of crisis. From its knowledge of rights, process and community resources, it may suggest avenues of advocacy the family has not considered.

The decision to care for an ill child at home requires regular reappraisal as free from guilt as possible. Lantos and Kohrman call this "renegotiation with dignity."[51] The medical establishment must not condemn parents who choose not to sacrifice their homes and lives to the best interests of the child.[52] At the same time, it must be prepared to activate social forces, such as child protection agencies, when families miss multiple appointments, fail to give regular medications, avoid therapeutic mental health services, or do not pursue the first steps toward arranging special education for the child.

Unfortunately, this sort of work is time-consuming and impractical in tertiary care in-patient units. Physicians are trained to be competent at technical decisions but are not as adept in situations, such as home care, where different values and personal choice assume a more important role.[53] Collaborative decision-making conflicts with traditionally prescriptive medical practices, threatens institutional paternalism, and challenges professionals' sense of responsibility. Still, hospitals and the providers who staff them must aim to make changes in the ways they practice, and they must involve others whose special expertise can complement their own when needed in order to fully understand and serve families taking on the burdens of home care.

Changes in Social Policy

The medical establishment and society in general have not been held accountable for their roles in expanding the problem of home care for children with chronic illness and disability. Kohrman wrote that society views as failures children who do poorly from a medical standpoint and has not yet elaborated a value system for "child–machine chimeras", those who depend upon technology to survive.[54] Constance Battle suggested that in "applauding the martyrdom" of mothers caring for neonatal intensive care unit survivors at home, society has attempted to absolve itself of guilt and any sense of responsibility to the family.[55]

Anthony Shaw wrote of critically ill newborns, "if society decides that the attempt must be made to salvage every human life, then society must provide the necessary funds and facilities to meet the continuing medical and psychological needs of these unfortunate children."[56] The "best interests of the child" standard on which this vitalist treatment imperative is based demands a societal commitment to provide resources to the family.[57] The strains of home care on the family are made worse by a lack of public services and community facilities.[58] At least two groups studying home care for ventilator-dependent children have called for the expansion of community-based extended care centers which can provide day-care and respite-care.[59]

Recent domestic policy planning has been focused less on society's obligation to look out for the well-being of families of children with chronic illness than on the fundamental right to medical care for all people. Most current health care reform proposals aim to assure adequate medical care for all children, regardless of their socioeconomic status. It is imperative that these proposals sustain or augment the level of services currently available under the best medical plans to families with children in home care, while extending insurability to all children. Writing of sick newborns, Lantos called for "a national policy that guarantees comprehensive follow-up care for handicapped neonatal intensive care unit survivors and guarantees adequate care for all pregnant women, and children."[60]

Society has done much in this century to bolster the rights of children with chronic illness and disability. It has asked parents simultaneously to assume overwhelming obligations in their children's home care and tolerate shrinking authority over the decisions that define these obligations. It is time to reassess the extent of these obligations from a moral perspective. Parents must be granted the opportunity to participate more fully in medical and educational planning for their children in the hospital, at school and at home. Until then, the burden of the inequity between parents' rights and choices and our expectations of them in home care will continue to be borne "All *on* the Family".

References

1. Lantos, J. and Kohrman, A. F. (1991). Ethical aspects of pediatric home care. In: *The Medically Complex Child: The Transition to Home Care*, edited by N. J. Hockstadt and D. M. Yost, Chur: Harwood. pp. 245–258.
2. Foster, S. and Hoskins, D. (1981). Home care of the child with a tracheostomy tube. *Pediatric Clinics of North America,* **28**:855–857; Ruben, R. J., Newton, L., Jornsay, D., Stein, R., Chambers, H., Liquori, J., and Lawrence, C. (1982). Home care of the pediatric patient with a tracheostomy. *Annals of Otology, Rhinology and Laryngology,* **91**:633–640.

3. Pinney, M. A., and Cotton, E.K. (1976). Home management of bronchopulmonary dysplasia. *Pediatrics,* **58**:856–859.
4. Spitz, R. A. (1946). Hospitalism: A follow-up report. *The Psychoanalytic Study of the Child,* **2**:113–117.
5. Oster, J. (1967). The child with Down's Syndrome (Mongolism), his parents and the community. *Acta Paediatrica Scandinavica, Supplement*, **172**:177–181; Oster, J. and Van dem Tempel, A. (1975). A 21-year psychosocial follow-up of 524 unselected cases of Down's Syndrome and their families. *Acts Pediatrica Scandinavica,* **64**:505–513.
6. Stone, N. D. (1973). The birth of a child with Down's Syndrome: A medico-social study of 31 children and their families. *Scottish Medical Journal,* **18**:182–187.
7. Stone, N. D. (1967). Family factors in willingness to place the mongoloid child. *American Journal of Mental Deficiency,* **72**:16–20.
8. Duff, R. S. and Campbell, A. G. M. (1973). Moral and ethical dilemmas in the special care nursery. *New England Journal of Medicine,* **289**(17):890–894.
9. Goldberg, A. I., Faure, E. A. M., Vaugh, C. J., Snarski, R. and Seleny, F. L. (1984). Home care for life-supported persons: An approach to program development. *J. Pediatr.,* **104**:785–795.
10. Goldberg, A. I. (1983). Home care a better life for ventilator-dependent people. *Chest,* **84**, p. 365.
11. Byrne, W. J., Halpin, T. C., Asch, M. J., Fonkalsrud, E. W. and Ament, M. E. (1977). Home total parenteral nutrition: An alternative approach to the management of children with severe chronic small bowel disease. *Journal of Pediatric Surgery,* **12**:359–366.
12. Cohen, C. B., Dubler, N. Genel, M., Moreno, J. P., Mundinger, M. and Post, S. (1987). "Section 6: Familial and social obligations to seriously ill and disabled children" In Imperiled Newborns. *Hastings Center Report* December 1987, 25–30.
13. Collopy, B., Dubler, N. and Zuckerman, C. (1990). The ethics of home care: Autonomy and accommodation. *Hastings Center Report, March/April 1990 Supplement*, 1–16.
14. Jennings, B., Callahan, D. and Caplan, A. L. (1988). Ethical challenges of chronic illness. *Hastings Center Report, February/March 1988*, 1–16.
15. Strobel, C. T. (1979). Home parenteral nutrition in children with Crohn's disease. *Gastroenterology,* **77**:1364; Burr, B. H., Guyer, B., Todres, I. D., Abrahams, B., and Chiodo, T. (1983). Home care for children on respirators. *New England Journal of Medicine,* **309**:1319–1323; Splaingarad, M. L., Frates, R. C., Harrison, G. M., Carter, R. E. and Jefferson, L. S. (1983). Home positive-pressure ventilation: Twenty years of experience. *Chest,* **84**:376–382; Wolfe, B. M., Beer, W. H., Hayashi, J. T., Halsted, C. H., Cannon, R. A. and Cox, K. L. (1983). Experience with home parenteral nutrition. *American Journal of Surgery,* **146**:7–12; Alcock, A. J. W., Hildes, J. A., Kaufert, P. A., Kaufert, J. M., and Bickford, J. (1984). Respiratory poliomyelitis: A follow-up study. *Canadian MedicalAssociation Journal,* **130**:1305–1310; Amarnath, R. P., Fleming, C. R., and Pernault, J. (1987). Home parenteral nutrition in chronic intestinal diseases: Its effect on growth and development. *Journal of Pediatric Gastroenterology and Nutrition,* **6**:89–95; Dwyer, E., Baker S. S., and Richardson, D. S. (1987). Home parenteral nutrition. In: *Pediatric nutrition: Theory and practice*, edited by R. J. Grand, J. L. Sutphen and W. H. Dietz, pp. 763–769. Boston: Butterworths; Quint, R. D., Chesterman, E., Crain, L. S., Winkelby, M. and Boyce, W. T. (1990). Home care for ventilator dependent children: Psychosocial impact on the family. *American Journal of Diseases of Children,* **144**:1238–1241; Bisset, W. M., Stapleford, P., Long, S., Chamberlain, A., Sokel, B. and Milia, P. J. (1992). Home parenteral nutrition in chronic intestinal failure. *Archives of Diseases in Childhood,* **67**:109–114.
16. Kaplan, J. E. and Moore, R. J. (1991). Legal rights and hurdles. In: *Children with Cerebral Palsy: A Parents' Guide*, edited by E. Geralis, pp. 297–332. U.S.: Woodbine House.
17. Downey, W. S. (1990). Public Law 99-457 and the clinical pediatrician. Part I: A description of the federal act and its predecessor. *Clinical Pediatrics,* **29**:158–161; Kaplan, J. E. and Moore, R. J. (1991). op. cit.
18. Juszczak, L. J. and Scheider, M. B. (1992). The chronically ill and disabled child in school. In *Pediatric Primary Care*, edited by R. A. Hoeckelman, pp. 640–642. St. Louis: Mosby.

19. Palfrey, J. S., Singer, J. D., Raphael, E. S. and Walker, D. K. (1990). Providing therapeutic services to children in special education placements: An analysis of the related services provision of PL 94-142 in five urban school districts. *Pediatrics,* **85**:518–525.
20. Ibid.
21. Thomas, G. H., Thomas, B. and Trachtenberg, S. W. (1993). Growing up with Patricia. *Pediatric Clinics of North America,* **40**:675–683.
22. Hobbs, N., Perrin, J. M. and Ireys, H. T. (1985). *Chronically Ill Children and Their Families*, pp. 102–126. San Francisco: Jossey-Bass.
23. Kohrman, A. F. and Diamond, L. (1986). Institutional and professional attitudes: Dilemmas for the chronically ill child. *Topics in Early Childhood Special Education,* **5**:82–91.
24. Groce, N. E. and Zola, I. K. (1993). Multiculturalism, chronic illness, and disability. *Pediatrics,* **92**:1048–1055.
25. Kohrman, A. F. and Diamond, L. (1984). Chronic illness and poverty: Children in double jeopardy. Presented at Bush Conference, Ann Arbor, MI.
26. Hobbs, N., Perrin, J. M. and Ireyes, H. T. (1985). op. cit.
27. Kohrman, A. F. and Diamond, L. (1986). op cit; Krener, P. and Adelman, R. (1988). Parent salvage and parent sabotage in the care of chronically ill children. *American Journal of Diseases of Children,* **142**:945–951; Fleischman, A. R. (1989). Ethical views and values. In: *Caring for Children with Chronic Illness: Issues and Strategies*, edited by R. E. K. Stein, pp. 87–100. New York: Springer; Groce, N. E. and Zola, I. K. (1993). op cit.
28. Lantos, J. and Kohrman, A. F. (1992). Ethical aspects of pediatric home care. *Pediatrics,* **89:** 920–924.
29. Goldstein, J., Freud, A. and Solnit, A. J. (1973). *Beyond the Best Interests of the Child*, pp. 13–14. New York: The Free Press (Macmillan).
30. Miezo, P. M. (1983). *Parenting Children with Disabilities: A Professional Source for Physicians and Guide for Parents*, pp. 20 and 66. New York: Marcel Dekker.
31. Drotar, D., Baskiewicz, A., Irvin, N., Kennell, J. and Klaus, M. (1975). The adaptation of parents to the birth of an infant with congenital malformation: A hypothetical model. *Pediatrics,* **56**:710–717; Jessop, D. J. and Stein, R. E. K. (1988). Essential concepts in the care of children with chronic illness. *Pediatrician,* **15**:5–12.
32. Sargent, J. and Liebman R. (1985). Childhood chronic illness: Issues for psychotherapists. *Community Mental Health Journal,* **4**:294–311; Jessop, D. J. and Stein, R. E. K. (1988). op. cit.
33. Olshansky, S. (1962). Chronic sorrow: A response to having a mentally defective child. *Social Casework,* **43**:190–193.
34. Sargent, J. and Liebman, R. (1985). op. cit. Cohen, C. B., Dubler, N., Genel, M., Moreno, J. P., Mundinger, M. and Post, S. (1987). op. cit; Kohrman, A. F. (1991). Psychological issues. In: *Delivering High Technology Home Care*, edited by M. J. Mehlman and S. J. Youngner, pp. 160–178. New York: Springer; Stein, R. E. K. (1992). Chronic physical disorders. *Pediatrics in Review,* **13**:224–229.
35. Kohrman, A. F. (1991). op. cit.
36. Battle, C. V. (1987). Beyond the nursery door: The obligation to survivors of technology. *Clinics in Perinatology,* **14**:417–427.
37. Frates, R. C., Harrison, G. M. and Splaingard, M. L. (1984). Home care for children on respirators. *New England Journal of Medicine,* **310**:1126–1127; Aday, L. A., Aitken, M. J. and Wegener, D. H. (1988). *Pediatric Home Care: Results of a National Evaluation of Programs for Ventilator Assisted Children.* University of Chicago, Center for Health Administration Studies, Continuing CHAS Research Series, No. 36. Chicago, Pluribus.
38. Kohrman, A. F. and Diamond, L. (1986). op. cit.
39. Bettelheim, B. (1987). *A Good Enough Parent: A Book on Child-Rearing*, p. 46. New York: Vintage.
40. Miezo, P. M. (1983). op. cit; Thomas, G. H., Thomas, B., and Trachtenberg, S. W. (1993). op. cit.
41. Battle, C. V. (1987). op. cit.

42. Kohrman, A. F. (1991). op. cit.
43. Collopy, B., Dubler, N. and Zuckerman, C. (1990). op. cit.
44. Feinberg, E. A. (1991). Ethical issues. In: *Delivering High Technology Home Care*, edited by M. J. Mehlman and S. J. Youngner, pp. 84–124. New York: Springer.
45. Lantos, J. and Kohrman, A. F. (1991). op. cit.
46. Cohen, C. B., Dubler, N. Genel, M., Moreno, J. P., Mundinger, M. and Post, S. (1987). op. cit.
47. Hardwig, J. (1990). What about the family? *Hastings Center Report, March/April 1990*, 5–10.
48. Lantos, J. and Kohrman, A. F. (1991). op. cit; Lantos, J. and Kohrman, A. F. (1992). op. cit.
49. Lantos, J. and Kohrman, A. F. (1992). op. cit.
50. Kohrman, A. F. (1991). op. cit.
51. Lantos, J. and Kohrman, A. F. (1991). op. cit.
52. Fleischman, A. R. (1989). op. cit.
53. Hobbs, N., Perrin, J. M. and Ireys, H. T. (1985). op. cit.
54. Kohrman, A. F. (1984). Pediatric home care: Ten-point agenda for the future. In: *Home Care for Children with Serious Handicapping Conditions.* Washington, D.C.: The Association for the Care of Children's Health; Kohrman, A. F. (1991). op. cit.
55. Battle, C. V. (1987). op. cit.
56. Shaw, A. (1973). Dilemmas of "Informed Consent" in Children. *New England Journal of Medicine,* **289**:885–890.
57. Fleischman, A. R. (1989). op. cit.
58. Jennings, B., Callahan, D. and Caplan, A. L. (1988). op. cit.
59. Aday, L. A., Aitken, M. J. and Wegener, D. H. (1988). op. cit. Quint, R. D., Chesterman, E., Crain, L. S., Winkelby, M. and Boyce, W. T. (1990). op. cit.
60. Lantos, J. (1987). Baby Doe five years later: Implications for child health. *New England Journal of Medicine,* **317**:444–447.

9 The Limits of the Physician's Duty to Treat

Jeffrey Burns and Robert Truog

Children's Hospital, Harvard Medical School,
Boston, Massachusetts 02115, USA

INTRODUCTION

It is self-evident that it is the patient who has the most at stake in any patient–physician encounter. The obligation to respect the wishes of the patient has a strong rational and compassionate foundation. Yet, many have recently noted an increasing controversy over who is to be the final arbiter in situations where a patient, or patient's surrogate, demands a specific diagnostic test or medical intervention that his or her physician believes is useless.[1–6] In these conflicts, how should the very compelling but competing claims of the patient for self-determination and of the physician for professional autonomy be balanced?

All physicians early in their training confront one end of the spectrum of this tension in medical care decision-making. The parent who insists on a prescription for an antibiotic when the physician has diagnosed a viral syndrome is familiar to nearly all pediatricians. The resolution of this conflict requires balancing such disparate issues as patient satisfaction, diagnostic accuracy, risk of allergic reaction, possible benefit (even if only placebo effect) and cost. Yet, even in the most difficult cases when relationships are strained and the air is charged with emotion, it is unusual in daily practice that some form of collaborative decision-making does not evolve. In those cases where agreement cannot be reached on the appropriate course of action, transfer of the patient to a willing physician usually removes (if not resolves) the conflict.

Clearly, patients or their surrogates do not have the right to demand *any* medical treatment they desire, and no professional tradition, ethical principle, or law, has ever required physicians to offer or accede to demands that are deemed medically inappropriate.[7] A physician would never amputate a limb on demand, treat a pneumonia with insulin, or provide similar therapies of no benefit because the patient insisted on it. For centuries many different societies have recognized this prerogative by conferring on the medical profession the exclusive authority to make judgments concerning medical care.

Moreover, no society could afford a universal health care system based on unchecked patient demands.[8] There are practical limits on the resources of any nation to provide health care, and our society is still searching for a consensus on the extent of any entitlement to health care. For most, this debate takes the form of defining the minimal level of services to which each citizen should be entitled. As amplified to life-saving or life-preserving care, a recent debate in the courts concerned whether a Californian health maintenance provider was obligated to cover bone marrow transplant therapy for a patient with breast cancer that was refractory to other forms of therapy. But, it is important to note that these are matters where there is no disagreement regarding the potential benefit, even if marginal, of the potential therapy. Rather, the issue is whether that benefit is worth the cost.

It is in the setting of critical care practice, however, (where life threatening conditions often preclude any resolution by transfer of care) that we are forced to confront the conflicting claims of patients and physicians to decide whether a treatment is beneficial or futile. Decisions on the limitation or withdrawal of life-sustaining care are always difficult for families and caregivers. But, in situations where a child is dying, who is the ultimate decision maker of when a therapy is useless or no longer indicated? Do physicians have a duty to respect a parent's agonizing need to do everything possible? Do patients or their surrogates have a right to therapy deemed medically worthless by their physician? Do physicians have a higher duty to respect professional judgment over patient autonomy, even if that means withdrawing life-support therapy?

Some trace the roots of this growing tension to the apparent ascendancy of patient autonomy in medical decision-making. This phenomenon, compounded by a medical tradition of trying all treatments that might be even marginally beneficial, has fostered what some see as an unrealistic sense of entitlement to unlimited medical care. Ingelfinger and others have argued that the profession is drifting dangerously close to abdicating fundamental principles of doctoring because too many physicians have a misguided understanding of ethical standards regarding respect for patient autonomy, and have adopted a 'vending machine' approach to medicine.[9] At its extreme, this unrestrained deference to patient autonomy reduces a physician to one who merely aligns an array of therapeutic options in front of the patient or family and then says, "go ahead and choose, it's your life." But, a proper understanding of doctoring would still preclude offering options to patients that their physicians consider to be without benefit, or harmful.

Others, notably Veatch and Spicer, argue that even if a surrogate's demand for care is "grossly inappropriate" and "deviates intolerably" from established standards, in cases of life-sustaining treatment the physician is obligated to continue. The only legitimate authority to assess the conflicting claims of patients and physicians, they believe, is "a socially legitimated authority" such as the judicial system.[10] Individual physician determination of when a therapy is medically futile is too open to value judgments, and therefore potential abuse, especially in cases of conflict over life-sustaining therapy. From this perspective, the state sanctioned privileges of licensure granted to the medical profession do not extend to unilaterally allowing physicians to impose their judgment of when a therapy is without benefit.

Despite these emerging opinions, there is no professional or societal consensus, or accumulation of case law, to define the limits of a physician's duty to treat. There are, however, two frequently discussed cases in the medical literature that highlight the competing values that surround this dilemma: Helga Wanglie and "Baby L".

The Helga Wanglie Case

Mrs. Helga Wanglie was an 85-year-old resident of a nursing home in January 1990 when she was transferred to the Hennepin County Medical Center in Minnesota, requiring emergency intubation and ventilator management for chronic bronchiectasis.[11] Five months later she was transferred to a chronic care facility after multiple attempts to wean her from mechanical ventilation had failed and she remained dependent on the ventilator. Before transfer she recognized her family and acknowledged occasional discomfort. One week after transfer, during another attempt to wean her from ventilator dependence, she suffered a cardiac arrest and was resuscitated. Shortly thereafter she was taken back to Hennepin County where she was found to be neurologically unresponsive. Over the next two months her husband, daughter and son insisted on continued treatment despite physicians' repeated recommendations to withdraw therapy that they deemed without benefit to the patient. (All her medical costs were covered by a combination of private insurance and Medicare funds). It is not clear whether Mrs. Wanglie ever stated her preferences concerning life-sustaining treatment before these events.

In November of the same year her physician told the family that he was no longer willing to continue to prescribe ventilator therapy. Mr. Wanglie, an attorney, rejected proposals to transfer the patient to another facility or to seek a court order mandating ventilator therapy. The Hennepin County Medical Center then petitioned the court to appoint an independent conservator to decide whether the ventilator was beneficial to the patient. While the court considered the matter, the family searched unsuccessfully for another facility that would care for Mrs. Wanglie. All facilities, including many with available beds, denied transfer, citing her poor rehabilitation potential. The trial court, however, in July 1991 appointed Mr. Wanglie as the conservator, stating he was best able to represent the patient's interest. Because no request to stop treatment had been made by the medical center, the trial court declined to speculate on the legality of such a request. Mrs. Wanglie died three days later of multisystem organ failure despite continuous aggressive therapy. The family stated the patient had received excellent care.

The Baby L Case

The most frequently cited pediatric case of a physician's refusal of a patient or surrogate demand for medical care involved the case of Baby L. As described by Paris *et al.*, Baby L was a 2-year-old girl at Children's Hospital in Boston when the controversy developed.[12] She was born to a 33-year-old mother, with three other children, weighing approximately 2 kg after a 36-week gestation. The pregnancy was complicated by fetal hydronephrosis and oligohydramnios in the third trimester. Thick meconium was noted on delivery, and she required aggressive resuscitation, with an APGAR score of 5 at ten minutes. Although she was successfully resuscitated and eventually weaned from mechanical ventilation, her neurological function was severely depressed with no responsiveness except to painful stimuli.

After 14 months of intensive care, including a tracheostomy and gastrostomy, she was discharged home with around-the-clock nursing care. Over the next 11 months she was hospitalized multiple times for recurrent aspiration pneumonia and sepsis, and suffered four cardiopulmonary arrests. At 23 months of age she continued to be responsive only to pain and her neurologic prognosis was deemed very poor.

At this time she was again admitted to Children's Hospital in a serious condition, again with a diagnosis of aspiration pneumonia, possibly needing mechanical ventilation if she deteriorated further. A meeting was convened by the medical team to consider the "advisability of reinstituting mechanical ventilation and cardiovascular support." The attendees included the primary physicians and nurses, as well as the chair of the hospital ethics committee, hospital counsel, and the chiefs of service. They unanimously agreed that "further medical intervention was not in the best interests of the patient," and "further intervention would subject the child to additional pain without affecting the underlying condition or ultimate outcome." The child's mother adamantly disagreed with this opinion.

Baby L. was able to be stabilized without mechanical ventilation. At the same time the hospital sought a facility that would be willing to accede to the mother's demands for intensive medical care if needed. The mother, meanwhile, contacted an attorney and arranged a hearing before a probate court. The judge apparently indicated a willingness to side with the mother's demands, but asked the attorney for the physicians what they would do if he issued an order for mechanical ventilation. The reply was that the physicians "would decline to participate in such an action," because it would violate their ethical obligation to the patient. The court then appointed a guardian for the child. A pediatric neurologist from another institution was asked by the guardian for an assessment of the child's condition and recommendations for care. The pediatric neurologist agreed with the assessment made by her physicians, including that she had severe neurological disability, and "was capable of experiencing pain, and that it was questionable whether she would survive, even with mechanical ventilation". Even so, the consultant neurologist was willing to accommodate the mother's demand for maximal medical therapy, and the child's care was transferred to another institution. Because there was no longer an unresolved conflict, the issue before the court was dismissed.

Several years later her first caregivers, who had advocated a limitation of medical therapy in the child's best interests, described her as still alive, although "blind, deaf, ... a quadriplegic ... and fed through a gastrostomy tube. She averages a seizure a day. Her pulmonary status has improved, but she continues to require intensive home nursing 16 hours a day. Her mental status remains that of a three month old infant."

The Unresolved Conflict

While frequently cited as prototypical cases for defining the limits of the physician's duty to treat, both cases were resolved in one manner or another before the courts had to issue an opinion. While the court in the Wanglie case did appoint Mr. Wanglie as the conservator, stating that he was best able to represent the patient's interest, this fell short of answering the question of whether and when a patient or surrogate can compel a physician to undertake or continue interventions deemed medically worthless.

There are other important ethical considerations raised by these two cases. The claim was made by Baby L's physicians that she was suffering. Does suffering change the limits of a physician's duty to treat? On another level, Mr. Wanglie, as an adult's surrogate, was claiming to present a "substituted judgment" for his wife. That is, on the basis of his intimate knowledge about Mrs. Wanglie's views when she was competent, he was purportedly making decisions based on what she would want under the specific circumstances. Baby L's mother, as is true for the surrogates of all young children, could not claim to act on the basis of substituted judgment. Most bioethicists and most courts have attempted to apply a different standard in making decisions for incompetent children, i.e., that of "best interests". However, reaching an adequate and practical definition of what exactly is meant by "best interests" has proven difficult for the bioethical and legal communities. The question arises as to whether the limits of a physician's duty to treat should be affected by the different justifications for the proxy's demand.

Despite these questions, the essential claim made by the physicians in both cases was that the intervention demanded would not affect the underlying condition or ultimate outcome. Therefore, with no medical indication, there was no obligation to provide the therapy. From this viewpoint, it ultimately did not matter whether the demand for therapy was made by the patient or by the patient's proxy. Similarly, apart from patient suffering, the physicians in these cases were arguing that there was a limit on their duty to treat when the intervention demanded was, in their judgement, without benefit.

There has been limited judicial review in the courts addressing this conflict. In 1986, the Massachusetts Supreme Court, in its decision in *Brophy v. New England Sinai Hospital*, ruled that patient Paul Brophy had the right to be free of unwanted life-sustaining medical treatment. They also ruled that physicians could not be required to act "if it would be contrary to their view of their ethical duty toward their patient". The court went on to say that the hospital and its staff "should not be compelled ... to act contrary to their moral and ethical principles, when such principles are recognized and accepted within a significant segment of the medical profession and hospital community."[13] In a similar light, the 1992 Virginia Commonwealth Health Care Decisions Act stated:

> Nothing in this article shall be construed to require a physician to prescribe or render medical treatment to a patient that the physician determines to be medically or ethically inappropriate. However, in such a case, if the physician's determination is contrary to the terms of an advanced directive of a qualified patient or the treatment decision of a person designated to make the decision under this article, the person shall make a reasonable effort to transfer the patient to another physician.

Both statements, while allowing for physician autonomy, again stop short of deciding whose views shall prevail given conflicting claims of patients and physicians regarding life-sustaining treatment.

This question has recently been addressed by England's Court of Appeal. In a 1992 unanimous decision, the court ruled in favor of a physician who stated he would not comply with a family's request to give a dying patient ventilator support if needed at some point to extend the patient's life. The ruling opinion stated in part that the courts, "should not require a medical practitioner ... to adopt a course of treatment which in the *bona fide* clinical judgment of the practitioner was contraindicated."[14]

Although there is little existing case law to guide patients and caregivers in defining the limits of a physician's duty to treat, it is clear that any adequate analysis of the conflicting claims must include the perspectives of the patient, the physician, and the norms of society.

PATIENTS' RIGHTS

The Rights of a Citizen to Health Care

Americans often speak loosely of a "right" to health care, yet the nature of such a right must be made clear. The notion of individual rights found in the American Constitution and Bill of Rights was inspired by the political philosophy of John Locke and Edmund Burke. They articulated the notion of people being sovereign over themselves, and having certain natural-born rights. While the nature and extent of these rights under our system of government have evolved and undergone different interpretations since then, most would agree that at a minimum a right defines a freedom. The right of free speech, to take a common example, is the freedom to engage in the expression of one's thoughts without undue coercion by another or the state. Philosophers and bioethicists further differentiate rights into negative rights and positive rights. A negative right is seen as the freedom from having something done *to* you. For instance, the right to privacy protects citizens from unlawful search and seizure. A positive right, on the other hand, is understood as a freedom to have something done *by* you. The implication behind a positive right is not only that a citizen has the right to some good or service, but that there is a consequent obligation on someone, often the state, to provide it.

The fundamental issue surrounding the debate on health care in late 20th century America is one of access and how much we are willing to pay for that access. While it is true that many Federal and state statutes require providers to deliver health care to eligible individuals without discrimination, there is no existing law that mandates a "right" to health care. The Constitution and Bill of Rights make no specific claim to such a notion. Physicians who staff emergency facilities and public hospitals are required by various regulations and laws to render care to all who may seek it, but this is in a strict sense only a "contract" between society (through the government) and physicians. Moreover, while medical care is increasingly a shared enterprise in which society acknowledges some obligation, (for example, through government-sponsored programs such as Medicaid and Medicare) coverage is not, at this time, universal and most Americans pay for their health care through privately managed insurance cooperatives.

But, it is important to note that issues of access are distinct from the dilemma over how to resolve the competing claims of a patient's demand for care that a physician determines is useless. The strength of a patient's claim to demand therapy that a physician deems worthless has less to do with the outcome of the debate over access to medical care deemed beneficial but costly, and more to do with determining the limits, if any, of respect for individual self-determination.

The Elevation of Patient Autonomy

The more powerful claim of the patient in conflicts over the usefulness of medical therapy is founded on the relatively recent ascendancy of the principle of respect for patient self-determination, or patient autonomy. Traditionally, the medical profession gave little weight to patient self-determination. Physicians routinely determined by themselves what information to withhold from a patient and what to disclose, when a therapy was useful, and when it was no longer indicated. This has been described as the paternalistic practice of medicine, which in recent years has given way to a dramatic shift toward patient autonomy. While this principle is not seen as providing a "right" to health care, respect for self-determination requires that patients be allowed the freedom to decide for themselves what is best, even if it is contrary to their doctor's opinion.

The ascendancy of the principle of respect for patient self-determination over physician paternalism is exemplified in the requirement for informed consent. The profound importance of this principle in health care decision-making is recognized and supported by the law and most of the medical establishment. It states that competent patients, or their surrogates, must be informed of any procedures or medical interventions to be undertaken by physicians. Moreover, the patient or surrogate has the right to refuse unwanted life-saving therapy, even if recommended by the physician.

However, there are clear limitations to an unbalanced approach to patient autonomy. No physician would feel compelled to amputate a healthy limb because a patient demanded it on the basis of respect for self-determination. But, many in the medical community do note a more subtle yet ethically and professionally perilous line of reasoning that results from unchecked adherence to the principle of patient autonomy. Smurl and Ingelfinger have been especially critical of physicians who they claim have accepted a misguided understanding of patient autonomy as non-interference, even to the point of doing what caregivers may otherwise consider medically and ethically unwise. The "glare of autonomy" has led, they argue, to the exaggerated expectation, even demand, by patients for health care services, and the abandonment by too many physicians of long held professional ideals, such as guiding desperately ill patients with crucial life choices.[15,16]

This sentiment was also expressed by the President's Commission for the Study of Ethical Problems in Medicine and Biomedical and Behavioral Research when they commented on the values underlying informed consent. While the Commission stated that patient self-determination is the most important ethical consideration relevant to resuscitation decisions, they also recognized another important ethical consideration, patient well-being, which requires the judgment of the physician. "Patients," they went on, "are not entitled to insist that health care practitioners furnish them services when to do so would violate either the bounds of acceptable practice or a professional's own deeply held moral beliefs or would draw on a limited resource on which the patient has no binding claim."[17] Respect for autonomy, to be consistent, requires not only respect for *patient* autonomy, but also respect for *professional* autonomy. The dilemma, of course, is how to balance these two claims when they conflict.

The ascendancy of a patient's claim to determine for himself or herself the appropriate course of medical care, even if he or she chooses to forego recommended life-saving therapy, is undisputed by bioethicists and the law. The foundation of this principle rests not on the national debate over the basic health care benefits due each citizen, but rather on respect for individual self-determination. Yet, while respect for patient autonomy logically requires reciprocal respect for professional autonomy, this alone does not establish that there are defensible limits to a physician's duty to treat. We must also explore the physician's obligations.

PHYSICIANS' DUTIES

Historical Foundations of the Duty to Treat

The foundation of any clinical encounter is that individuals seek a doctor's care because they think they need help, and physicians with their specialized training and knowledge assess the situation and determine whether their skills can be beneficial. Deciding what is beneficial must reflect a balance between the competing demands of the physician's professional charge. On the one hand, physicians are obliged to avoid harm (acts of omission) in their attempts to help. Yet, physicians are also obligated to do good (acts of commission) by intervening to save a life or treat an injury.

If a physician's duties were not defined by the accepted ideals of the profession, then individual practitioners would not have to adhere to certain standards, but only to personal beliefs. However, medicine, like other professions, according to Reed,[18] is distinguished by several characteristics: (1) The profession is in possession of a circumscribed and valuable body of knowledge. (2) The members of the profession determine the profession's standards of competence and expertise. (3) The profession is given authority to license practitioners by the State, with licensing and admission boards made up largely of members of the profession. (4) The profession has a code of ethics or standards that govern practice. (5) The profession is largely free of lay control, with its practitioners exercising a high degree of autonomy.

While these characteristics are reflective of the medical profession today, determining the essential obligation and norms of the modern physician–patient relationship is less clear. The origins of a physician's professional duty, for instance, are often told. Yet, attempts to ground a modern professional ethic in historic precedent are not possible, for there has been no consistent professional tradition.

It is often quoted that Hippocrates urged physicians in the *Epidemics* to "Declare the past, diagnose the present, foretell the future; practice these acts. As to disease, make a habit of two things — to help, or at least do no harm."[19] The central commitment flowing from this tradition is understood to be one of beneficence, to use one's special skills to benefit the sick. Yet, Hippocrates also recognized that medicine had its limits. In *The Art* he wrote, "I will define what I conceive medicine to be. In general terms, it is to do away with the sufferings of the sick, to lessen the violence of their diseases, and to refuse to treat those who are overmastered by their diseases, realizing that in such case's medicine is powerless."[20] The Hippocratic conception of the professional duty thus emphasizes two commitments: first, to benefit the patient by providing therapy for injury and disease; and, second, to avoid harm at all times, especially when there is no reasonable prospect for success. While such a perception of the physician's obligations would seem to support a limit on the doctor's duty to treat, the ensuing historic ideal did not always give equal weight to the two commitments.

The behavior of notable physicians into the Middle Ages can best be characterized by the avoidance of self-sacrifice. For instance, little attempt was made to treat patients during the great pandemics of the time out of concern for the physician's own safety, and to a lesser degree because the doctor's believed their efforts to be powerless against the disease processes at hand. When the plague ravaged Rome in 166 AD. Galen admitted to fleeing the city, as did Thomas in 1655 when the plague struck London. Not only was this true of the famous physicians of the day, but of the profession as a whole. Medieval chroniclers also detailed how nearly all the physicians in Venice fled in terror when the plague befell that city.[21]

On the other hand, the relatively more recent historical record, and the ideal type that persists in the folklore of medicine, is one of an emphasis on beneficence as the overriding professional duty. Many stories that persist from the cholera pandemics in the 17th and 18th centuries, the influenza pandemic of 1918, and the polio epidemic in the 1950's before the Salk vaccine, champion physicians who cared for patients at great personal risk, and despite the fact that cures were impossible for infections of that time. The shift toward a commitment to patients' well being, despite the futile therapeutic regimens of the time, can be seen as early as the first AMA Code of Ethics in 1847. It instructed physicians that "... when pestilence prevails, it is their duty to face the danger, and to continue their labors for the alleviation of the suffering, even at the jeopardy of their own lives."[22] The emphasis from this era of the medical tradition, then, is that a physician's duty extends beyond providing care that may be curative, and this would allow an interpretation of professional obligations that places no limit on the duty to treat.

Recent professional codes are as ambiguous as the historical record in declaring the fundamental duty of a physician. The current American Medical Association Principles of Medical Ethics, in Section 6, reads, "A physician shall, in the provision of appropriate patient care, except in emergencies, be free to choose whom to serve, with whom to associate, and the environment in which to provide medical service."[23] Many bioethicists accept this provision and speak of the physician–patient relationship as one of a "contract between free and equal moral agents". This characterization of the relationship would seem to lessen the emphasis on the categorical nature of the professional duty, allowing more weight to the physician's discretion in determining when medicine is powerless, and the physician's duties limited. Arras has noted that the language of the current AMA Code of Ethics was introduced in 1957, a period when medicine appeared to have succeeded in controlling pandemics of one etiology or another, thus supporting an environment of contractualism.[24] Recent debates over the ethical obligations of physicians in providing informed consent and in caring for patients with the HIV infection, however, have forced a reappraisal of the physician–patient relationship.

The Ethical Foundation of the Duty to Treat

The struggle to define the balance of decision-making authority in the physician–patient relationship has prompted many bioethicists to describe the various manifestations of the relationship. There have been many proposals for a preferred model, or ideal type, that fill a continuum from the *Paternalistic* (also known as the parental or priestly) model, where the physician acts as the patient's guardian and determines what course of therapy is best, to the *Informative* (also described as the consumer, engineering, or scientific) model, where the physician presents the facts to the patient but leaves all the decisions to the latter.[25]

The informative model as the ideal type has gained increasing predominance in the past 20 years. Many cite the endorsement for this model in the law, beginning with the landmark case of *Canterbury v Spence* in 1972. In this case on informed consent the U.S. Court of Appeals, District of Columbia Circuit, ruled "... it is the prerogative of the patient, not the physician, to determine for himself the direction in which his interests seem to lie." [26] This sentiment is also embodied in the New York State *Uniform Rights of the Terminally Ill Act,* which in 1987 declared that the "... Act authorizes an adult person to control decisions regarding administration of life-sustaining treatment."[27]

Some have argued for a move to a middle ground through such notions as the *Collegial* or *Deliberative* model, for which the physician and patient are seen as equal colleagues negotiating together to define a mutually agreeable goal. Others strive for a middle ground model, but place more emphasis on a contractual foundation to the relationship ("free and equal moral agents") in which the physician has a fiduciary obligation to act in the patient's interests as the patient defines it, but also has autonomy in choosing when and how to serve.

In a pluralistic society, however, there is no agreement on what is the ideal type for the physician–patient model. The shifting norms of patient rights and physician obligations leave unsettled the question of who is to be the final arbiter on the limits of a doctor's duty to treat. Nevertheless, it is an inescapable dimension of medical care that in most respects it is the physician who determines the therapeutic options that are to be considered. If a treatment is not judged to be beneficial to the situation at hand, then the patient is generally not informed about it. One of the ethical challenges in shared medical decision-making, therefore, is to provide an objective set of standards to be used in assessing what is material to the decision an autonomous patient is entitled to make.

Futility as a Justification for a Limit on the Physician's Duty to Treat

Few terms in medical ethics have provoked as much controversy as "futility". Futility is inherently an elusive concept, since there is no universally agreed-upon objective of medical care, nor is there agreement on the criteria that should be used to evaluate outcomes of that care. It has been noted that the word futility has its origins in the Latin word "futilis", which means "leaky". In Greek mythology the daughters of Danaus were condemned in Hades to draw water in leaky sieves, and thus their labors were useless.

In recent medical practice, the concept of futility has been advanced by some physicians as a purportedly objective means of limiting medical therapy based on a professional judgment and despite patient or surrogate demands to the contrary. Proponents of futility have advanced this notion because, as Truog has noted, "it offers a reason to limit therapy without the need to define a fair procedure for allocating scarce resources. This approach allows treatments to be denied on the grounds that they are simply not indicated, apart from the matter of cost ..."[28] In essence, invoking the claim of futility licenses professional judgment to take precedence over patient autonomy in decision-making.

Several approaches to futility have been proposed, but the interpretation that has provoked the most discussion recently is that put forward by Schneiderman and colleagues.[29] Futility, Schneiderman argues, provides an objective basis for physicians to make a professional judgment to withhold or withdraw medical therapy deemed inappropriate, without subjecting such a decision to patient approval. This is to be distinguished from the subjective attitude of hopelessness. Hopelessness is fundamentally a personal value judgment that is open to each physician's interpretation and potentially subject to abuse. Schneiderman and colleagues argue that their meaning of futility is based on specific criteria designed to overcome this subjectivity. Futility in this sense has both a quantitative and qualitative component.

In the quantitative sense, futility is any effort to achieve a result that by experience or reasoning is "highly improbable". Although "highly improbable" is a statistical judgment which implies an objective determination, Schneiderman acknowledges that in a strict sense this is rarely possible. The data upon which physicians prognosticate is almost never derived from prospective comparisons of precisely controlled and identically matched cohorts of patients with the peculiar problems of the individual patient to which the results are to be generalized. Since the ideal conditions for determining probability will never be present, they argue instead for another standard upon which to base a quantitative notion of highly improbable. If no successes in 100 trials of a particular therapy are observed, then this data can serve as a "point estimate of the probability of treatment success." While they admit that 100 observations of no benefit do not support the claim that the treatment never works, they are sufficient grounds for the physician to make a professional judgment that the outcome of such therapy is so unlikely to produce the goal intended that it can fairly and rationally be judged as futile.

The qualitative notion of futility, by their definition, is understood to be "any treatment that merely preserves permanent unconsciousness or that fails to end total dependence on intensive medical care ... or continued biologic life without conscious autonomy." Schneiderman and colleagues go on to express their judgment that a "patient has no right to be sustained in a state in which he or she has no purpose other than mere vegetative survival: the physician has no obligation to offer this option or services to achieve it."

Critics of the meaning of futility as put forth by Schneiderman and colleagues cite two major deficiencies. First, attempting to wrap the concept in objectivity by invoking such a quantitative definition is based on an overconfident reliance on the accuracy of clinical trials. Second, critics charge that the value judgments of physicians are no more inherently valid than those of patients.

For instance, although medicine has achieved remarkable advances in diagnosis and therapy based on the scientific method of reductionism, our notion of "effective therapy" for a given disease process is based on the often imperfect method of clinical trials. The tradition of most journals has been to enthusiastically report when something works, but less recognized by the medical community has been the inadequate basis for many studies that report a result of no benefit for a particular intervention. Biostatisticians and epidemiologists have recently warned that a high percentage of clinical trials from major medical journals that reported negative results (e.g., those that found no difference between the treatments that were studied) could have missed an important difference in therapies because inadequate numbers of subjects were evaluated. Many of these studies actually showed trends suggesting that a treatment worked, but the authors concluded that the therapy was no different from control simply because, statistically, they could not reject the null hypothesis. Only 2 of 93 papers from breast cancer trials, according to Mosteller and colleagues, contained a discussion of statistical power. The "power of a study" was a frequently overlooked component of clinical trials until recently, but it is critical in studies that find no difference between the test and control arms. It is defined as the probability that the trial will detect a treatment effect of a particular difference for a particular number of experimental subjects. The higher the power, the better the chances of finding the treatment benefit, if it is there. Thus for Schneiderman to propose a quantitative notion based on 100 consecutive treatment failures presupposes an accuracy in clinical trial results that is open to serious question based on expert review of the existing literature in a variety of fields.

Moreover, as Truog noted, even excluding clinical trial results, psychological research has shown that the tendency to remember cases that are unusual or bizarre predisposes physicians to make decisions on the basis of their experiences with unusual cases.[30] Thus, estimating the efficacy of a particular therapy based on personal memory is an unreliable method of applying previous experience to the peculiarities of the present case.

The second major criticism is that the qualitative notion of futility they propose is intrinsically value-laden. Ours is a pluralistic society in which people espouse deeply held, often incommensurate values. The mother of Baby L, and Mr. Wanglie, rejected the conclusion that therapies that continued biologic life without consciousness or with dependence on intensive medical care should be considered worthless. These views are understandable and defensible. It is also clear that physicians do not possess any super-human ability through unique personal gifts or professional training to divine the priority of health-related values over other values. This is not to state that the physician's values are of less merit than the patient's in these matters and therefore of less weight; but, it is to question whether the physician's value preferences should be revered as unilaterally determinative.

BALANCING PATIENTS' RIGHTS AND PHYSICIANS' DUTIES

The relatively recent move toward the primacy of patient autonomy and the corresponding shift away from unregulated physician paternalism are based on the self-evident truth that it is the patient who has the most at stake in the decision-making process. Combined with the inconsistent tradition of the medical profession and the difficulties in reaching unassailable objective standards to define a therapy as futile, can we conclude that either the patient's or the physician's views should prevail in conflict involving life-sustaining care? Or are the opposing claims both deserving of respect and thus both obliged to accept a process of adjudication and balancing?

It is impractical in the modern age of technology-based medical care for any patient or surrogate to be fully abreast of the multitude of decisions, choices, and options considered consciously or unconsciously by physicians. The abundance of information that is routine in any medical encounter, let alone that accumulated in complex cases, requires synthesis, interpretation, and selective emphasis based on years of training and experience. This fact of the information age means that physicians are continually making judgments on what therapy is worthwhile. Moreover, restricting physicians to determining empirical fact, issuing technical advice, and potentially overriding their own values if demanded by the patient, is not only impractical but unwise.

If physicians become tied to a sense of uncritical compliance, and not to a sense of professional judgment, it will diminish not only the profession, but the quality of care and comfort that desperately ill patients need. Physicians, it has been noted, could quickly lose a sense of purpose and dignity if their values were always overridden by their patients' demands. While at first glance concern for physician ideals and dignity may seem trivial in comparison to ensuring the primacy of patient autonomy in decision-making regarding life-sustaining therapy, there is shortsightedness in forcing professionals to act against their best judgment. Imagine the cumulative loss of purpose that surgeons would experience if they were compelled to undertake patient-demanded operations that they deemed useless. Similarly, what would be the long-term impact on the outlook and sense of purpose of critical-care physicians and nurses if they were forced to maintain technological immortality on bodies in their units?

The law, too, has recognized the negative consequences of allowing patients' demands to always prevail. In *Brophy v. New England Sinai Hospital* the Supreme Judicial Court of Massachusetts upheld the right of the hospital's medical staff to refuse to participate in an act that violated their moral and ethical principles. It ruled that there is nothing in the law "which would justify compelling medical professionals ... to take active measures which are contrary to their view of their ethical duty toward their patients."[31] At some level society also seems to recognize this, for the ideal characterization of a physician that persists in our popular culture is not that of an automaton who efficiently provides facts and unquestionably does other's bidding. Rather, it is of a person who brings wisdom, judgment, compassion and insight into the physician–patient relationship.

It is the legitimate prerogative of physicians to place some limit on their duty to treat, even in cases of life-sustaining care and despite patient or surrogate demands to the contrary. The New York State Task Force on Life and the Law also expressed support for this position when they stated, "Physicians currently have no duty to provide treatment that is futile in the narrow sense of the term — treatment that will not achieve any identified medical benefit, including the prolongation of life."[32] A strict duty to treat, based on the notion that patients have a right to demand specific therapies has never been established. No professional code, ethical principle, or law has ever required doctors to accede to patient's wishes upon demand. Moreover, to do so would lead to a significant violation of professional dignity and purpose that would, in our judgment, far outweigh the marginal benefits of yielding to patient autonomy.

Ultimately, the decision by a physician to refuse requested life-sustaining therapy that is deemed useless comes down to a judgment of what is in the patient's best interests. Distinguishing an improper imposition of a physician's values on a patient and a proper commitment to a patient's best interests will never be easy. All such judgments are, fundamentally, value-laden. This does not mean, however, that they are wrong. All pediatricians recognize that there are rare instances in which it is the physician's obligation to override a parent's wishes, no matter how well intended. Parents of a child with life-threatening sepsis do not have a right to demand a therapy such as prayer without medical intervention. No physician would feel compelled to follow such demands. Indeed, it would be the physician's professional obligation to override the parent's demands in such a case.

Similarly, it is inconsistent with accepted medical practice to subject any patient to worthless and harmful therapy. While the goals of the physician–patient relationship have varied in the history of medicine, a persistent theme has been that it should entail some degree of beneficence. Inflicting useless, burdensome, or harmful treatment in the service of autonomy demonstrates a disrespect for the dignity and worth of the patient. While it is impossible, because of disagreements on statistical certainty and the value of outcomes, to specify the level of medical certitude necessary to make such a judgment, it is nevertheless a decision within the domain of professional authority.

Just as there are circumstances where physicians should intervene when parents refuse life-saving therapy for a treatable disease, so too are there circumstances where physicians may refuse to accede to demands for disproportionately burdensome life-preserving care. Both decisions involve a professional judgment that is in part value-laden. But, traditionally, our professional training and societal norms have authorized us to take responsibility for the former. Now, we must promote recognition of our authority to make the most appropriate decisions about the latter.

Since the right of self-determination is appropriately accorded such great moral significance by society and the medical profession, the rare circumstance of a physician refusing to treat in opposition to a patient's demand must follow strict procedural safeguards. Essential features of such a process would first entail the development by the profession, or affiliated societies, of a clear policy on the sequence to be followed when a physician determines a limit on the duty to treat. If a conflict between the physician and the patient cannot be resolved in the usual manner, or by transfer of the patient to another physician or institution, consultants, preferably from another institution, should be called to review the facts of the case and render an opinion. The institution's ethics committee, or equivalent, should also be asked to review the case, help delineate the pertinent values in contention, and make recommendations. The entire process requires as much openness as respect for patient confidentiality will allow. Additionally, the profession, or at least the particular institutions involved, should seek judicial review and financially support legal costs for both sides. This approach will help to ensure procedural fairness by counterbalancing the inherent advantages of the institution and medical team over the patient or family, and provide a forum so that the patient's goals for therapy are openly addressed. It would also demonstrate professional responsibility on an issue that will always be contentious.

The Society of Critical Care Medicine has begun such a process. Through its Ethics Task Force, and in response to concerns raised by many of its members, a guideline was drafted, debated, and then approved that states that patients in a persistent vegetative state may be refused admission to intensive care units at the sole discretion of the intensivist.[33] This position is currently before the leadership council of the society. The next step in the process is formal adoption by the Society of Critical Care Medicine at large. Based on the safeguards already articulated, an appropriate sequence before making this an accepted practice would be for the Society of Critical Care Medicine, or an institution or medical staff adopting the policy, to seek judicial review of initial cases.

These extraordinary steps in the physician–patient relationship, while fortunately rare, are to be undertaken with great caution, and only after having followed an open review process. Technological advances may lead to increasing conflicts along these lines. If, however, physicians remember that autonomy is best served by offering choices that are medically and ethically reasonable, then patients will receive truly caring therapy.

References

1. Brett, A. S. and McCullough, L. B. (1986). When patients request specific interventions: defining the limits of the physician's obligation. *N. Eng. J. Med.,* **315**:1347–1351.
2. Paris, J. J., Crone, R. K. and Reardon, F. (1990). Physicians' refusal of requested treatment: the case of Baby L. *N. Eng. J. Med.,* **322**:1012–1014.
3. Miles, S. H. (1991). Informed demand for "non beneficial" medical treatment. *N. Eng. J. Med.,* **325**:512–515.
4. Blackhall, L. J. (1987). Must we always use CPR? *N. Eng. J. Med.,* **317**:1281–1215.
5. Engelhardt, H. T. (1979). Rights to health care: a critical appraisal. *J. Med. Philos.,* **4**:113–117.
6. Paris, J. J., Schreiber, M. D., Statter, M., Arensman, R. and Siegler, M. (1993). Beyond autonomy; physicians' refusal to use life-prolonging extracorporeal membrane oxygenation. *N. Engl. J. Med.,* **329**:354–357.
7. Schneiderman, L. J., Jecker, N. S. and Jonsen, A. R. (1990). Medical futility: its meaning and ethical implications. *Ann. Intern. Med.,* **112**:950.
8. Thurow, L. C. (1984). Learning to say "No". *N. Eng. J. Med.,* **311**:1569–1572.
9. Ingelfinger, F. J. Arrogance (1980). *N. Eng. J. Med.*, **303**:1507–1511
10. Veatch, R. M. and Spicer, C. M. (1992). Medically futile care: the role of the physician in setting limits. *Am. J. Law. Med.,* **18**:15–36.
11. Miles, S. H. (1991). op. cit. p. 513.
12. Paris, J. J. *et al.*, (1990). op. cit. p. 1012–1014.
13. Brophy v. New England Sinai Hospital, 389 Mass., 417, 497 N.E. 2d 626 (1986).
14. Re J. (a minor). Court of Appeal. 10 June, 1992. Lord Chief Justice Donaldson. Cited in: Kerreth R. British judges cannot order doctors to treat. *Hastings Centre Report* (1992), **22**(4):3–4.
15. Smurl, J. F. (1990). Point-counterpoint: physicians' refusal of requested treatment. *J. Perinatol,* **10**, p. 410.
16. Ingelfinger, F. J. (1980). op. cit. p. 1507.
17. President's Commission for the Study of Ethical Problems in Medicine and Biomedical and Behavioral Research. Deciding to forego life-sustaining treatment: a report on the ethical, medical and legal issues in treatment decisions. Washington, D.C.: U.S. Government Printing Office, 1983, pp. 41–46.
18. Reed R. R. and Evans D. (1987). The Deprofessionalization of Medicine. *JAMA,* **258**:3279–3282.
19. Hippocrates. Epidemics. In: *Hippocrates*, trans. Jones W. Cambridge, Massachusetts: Harvard University Press, 1923, **I**, p. 165.
20. Ibid., The Art, **II**, p. 193.
21. Zugar, A. and Miles, S. H. (1987). Physicians, AIDS, and occupational risk: historic traditions and ethical obligations. *JAMA*, **258**:1924–1928.
22. Ibid., Historic Traditions, p. 1926.
23. American Medical Association, Principles of Medical Ethics. 1980. In: *Biomedical Ethics.* (1991). Mappes T. A., Zembaty J. S., (eds.) New York: McGraw-Hill, p. 53.
24. Arras, J. D. (1988). AIDS and the duty to treat. *Hastings Center Report,* **18**:10–18.
25. Emanuel, E. J. and Emanuel, L. L. (1992). Four models of the physician-patient relationship. *JAMA*, **267**:2221–2226.
26. Robinson, S. W. (1972). Opinion in Canterbury v. Spence. In: *Biomedical Ethics.* Mappes, T. A., Zembaty, J. S. (eds.) New York: McGraw-Hill, pp. 88–91.
27. Ibid., p. 89.
28. Truog, R. D., Brett, A. S. and Frader, J. (1992). The problem with futility. *N. Eng. J. Med.,* **326**:1560–1563.
29. Schneiderman, L. Y. *et al.*, (1990). op. cit. p. 949–54.
30. Truog, R. D. *et al.*, (1992) op. cit. p. 1562.
31. Brophy v New England Sinai Hospital (1986). op. cit.

32. Medical Futility: Defining the Limits of the Duty to Treat, Chapter 14: When Others Must Choose: Deciding for Patients Without Capacity. Report of the New York State Task Force on Life and the Law, New York: The Task Force (1992) 203.
33. Society of Critical Care Medicine Ethics Committee, Consensus Statement in the Triage of Critically Ill Patients *JAMA,* (1994), **271**:1200–1203.

10 Bridging the Tensions Between Care and Cure

Cindy Hylton Rushton

Johns Hopkins Children's Center, 600 N. Wolfe St, Baltimore, Maryland 21205, USA

INTRODUCTION

Providing care to critically or terminally ill infants and children is challenging both for families and for health care providers. Treatment decisions are often made under conditions of great uncertainty and urgency. At times, patients and their families and health care providers are strangers to one another when they are thrust into an intense, vulnerable relationship with each other. Decision-making under such conditions is a complex process that is influenced by the way parents and professionals view their respective worlds.

Everyone sees the world through his or her own social, scientific and value frameworks. Each views the world through different lenses; each uses different maps to guide the way they look at the world, the way they perceive reality and the way they structure knowledge. Their view of the world guides what they pay attention to and what they discount, and how they use the information available to them. Even when individuals examine "the same world", they do so for a variety of purposes, from a variety of vantage points, and each will produce a different picture that is no more or less valid than the other.

The various professionals who care for critically ill children and their families may also have different views of their respective worlds. Medicine and nursing, for example, share common values and goals. Both are committed to promoting the patient's well-being. Each discipline, however, interprets patient well-being based upon the profession's values, knowledge base, social norms, and unique sense of concern. These dimensions of the profession provide a map to guide inquiry, behavior, and decision-making.[1] The profession's map alerts its members to what is relevant to achieving a particular value or goal and points to how to achieve it.[1,2]

As compassionate caregivers, physicians, for example, have altruistic motives in caring for their patients; but, they may also be guided by the imperative of technology to repair or enhance the child's anatomy or physiology principally because it is technically and logistically feasible. Often their goal is to cure the patient's problem or enhance his or her level of functioning to the greatest extent possible.

Nurses often share similar values about prolonging life but by contrast, they may view the same child's care in a different context. Their assessment of the child's treatment may be influenced by their intimate understanding of the child's unique responses to therapy and to an evolving appreciation of the parent's values, goals and hopes for their child. Their goal is to optimize the patient's and family's responses to the disease and to promote individualized coping and adaptation to their situation. This does not mean that one perspective is superior to the other, only that each discipline uses different maps to guide their attention and concerns.

These differences in views of the world invite moral conflicts between families and health care professionals. Moral conflicts arise when competing moral considerations underlie various treatment alternatives. The potential for moral conflict escalates in proportion to the uncertainty surrounding the care of critically ill infants and children.[3] Conflicts are further complicated by the following: poor or confusing communication between families and care providers, inadequate informed consent, lack of collaboration among health care team members and/or parents, inconsistency in the decision-making process that results in poorly defined treatment parameters, and decisions made by default.[4,5]

In general, there are two prominent views of the care of patients and their families: the perspectives of cure and of care. In this chapter, the assumptions of the perspective of cure and care will be explored. Some of the conflicts that arise when these perspectives clash will be discussed and strategies for blending the perspectives of care and cure will be offered.

ASSUMPTIONS OF THE CURE PERSPECTIVE

Cure is generally the guiding value in the treatment of patients. In the acute-care setting in particular, the focus is on the technologic support of body functions. For example, when a young child admitted to the hospital with a vague diagnosis of lethargy, fever, and anorexia acutely deteriorates, the goal of intervention is to support his body systems until a cause for the dysfunction is identified. This may involve the use of ventilators, hemodynamic monitoring, and a variety of medications.

Given this allegiance to cure, success is measured by the percentage of survivors and the length of life. How that life is lived is of secondary concern. When various treatment options are considered, the benefits of survival may overshadow the attendant burdens. The pursuit of the underlying cause of the illness may result in prolonged mechanical ventilation, numerous invasive diagnostic or therapeutic procedures, isolation, and diminished opportunities for meaningful interaction. Despite this, the goal remains the preservation of the child's life. This creates a high threshold for tolerating burdens or complications in order to achieve cure or survival. In the extreme, the cure perspective supports attempting to save life at all costs in every instance. This means that if a treatment holds even a remote chance of saving life, it must be tried.

The cure perspective is consistent with the prevailing scientific paradigm. Therefore, the treatment of sick patients is guided by an effort to isolate a specific cause or set of causes in order to account for the observed effect on the patient's anatomy, physiology or psyche. Disease is understood in terms of deviations from physiologic norms. For cases viewed from such a perspective, a number of specialists may be called to identify a cause that might lead to an effective treatment. Each may focus his or her attention on a specific organ system and on the anatomic, physiologic or biochemical indicators of that system's functioning. To this end, the patient's symptoms and responses become "medicalized"; they are transformed into medical terms and the illness experience is molded and filtered through the lenses of medicine. The reality is cast in terms of physiologic, anatomic, or psychological causal matrices.[6] It is the numbers that count: the intake, the output, the weight, the blood gases, the vital signs, etc. From this view it is assumed that diagnosis will lead to treatment, and that treatment will, eventually, lead to cure.

From the cure perspective, truth is learned through science. Although particular scientific communities embrace certain facts, findings, and rules of evidence and inference, they are unified in their belief that for scientific knowledge to be useful it must be reliable and valid. To be reliable it must be public, universalizable, and free of subjective biases such as individual beliefs, values, or attitudes. Such an approach depends on a "value-free" method of collecting facts and reaching conclusions. Providers must maintain a detached attitude in order to accurately interpret patient data. Hence, rationality, objectivity, and logic are central to decision-making.[7]

The search for knowledge is a powerful motivator for continuing the quest toward a greater understanding of disease and patient responses to treatment. With the ever-increasing body of knowledge about the human body and the explosion of technology that has paralleled its growth, there is increasingly an imperative to use technology to achieve diagnosis, treatment, and, ultimately, cure. This is evident in tertiary acute-care settings, particularly intensive care units.

However, there may also be other motivations for adopting the cure perspective. Allegiance to the cure perspective may also be guided by a value that life in any form is valuable and therefore ought to be preserved regardless of other factors. Such a vitalist view would lead one to pursue whatever means are medically possible to prolong life. Another motivation may be that professional competence and success is determined by patient survival and to lose a patient to death is viewed as a failure of skill, knowledge, or judgement. This may result in professionals embracing the heroic challenge to overcome the forces of disease by employing whatever means are necessary.

ASSUMPTIONS OF THE CARE PERSPECTIVE

The focus of the care perspective is on providing holistic care. The constitutive dimensions of the human being are viewed in the context of the whole person, rather than as independent, isolated systems. Treatment of a dysfunction within a body system, for example, the renal system, focuses not only on the manipulation of the patient's fluids and blood chemistries but on the impact of the dysfunction on other body systems and the patient's overall functioning and quality of life. The body's dysfunctions must be viewed, understood and treated within the content of the mind and spirit of the person.

Holistic care encompasses caring for and about another by rendering needed services and by attending to the person's physical, emotional, and spiritual well-being. A holistic approach to care recognizes that health cannot be guaranteed by curing an illness or eradicating disease. Rather, the goal is to enable the patient, family, and significant others to adjust to the changes in health in their own unique way. From this view, survival and cure become incidental rather than primary. Healing becomes the ultimate goal rather than focusing on cure as the ultimate outcome. Interventions then are directed toward maximizing the control exerted by the patient and family. In this way, the patient's sense of personhood, self-worth, and dignity are advanced. This ideology is based on such humanistic criteria as quality-of-life or coping ability, rather than a disease classification approach.[8]

From the perspective of care, truth is learned through the lived experience. Truth is multidimensional and embedded in the context of individual lives and relationships and evolves over time through dialogue and interaction.[9] Reciprocity between the individual, other human beings and the environment creates the context for the lived experience. The interests of children, for example, cannot be separated from the context of their families. Such reciprocity also includes health care professionals who create the context for the illness experience. The perspective of care, therefore, insists that a meaningful, interactive relationship among patient and family and health care providers is necessary for effective advocacy and treatment.

Moral uncertainty is viewed as a reality of the lived experience and not as an impediment to moral agency. An acceptance of the ambiguity surrounding illness and disease diffuses the need to pursue every avenue possible to eradicate the uncertainty. For example, when a diagnosis is unclear but multiple organ systems are failing it may be unnecessary from a care perspective to pursue further invasive diagnostic tests that are unlikely to alter the patient's eventual outcome.

The care perspective supports efforts to assist patients and/or their families to find unique meaning or purpose in their living or their dying and to assist them to realize goals that facilitate the experience of such meaning. For example, a terminally ill child with cancer and his parents may value comfort, optimal function despite limitations, and being in their home environment. During the dying process they can be supported to pursue treatments that are aimed at relieving pain and symptoms and that promote family integrity rather than pursing an experimental chemotherapeutic regimen.

For such a personalized perspective, scientific facts may have secondary relevance to determining the proper course of action. The choices may not be simply right or wrong, but may have more to do with the implications of each option for the character of the persons involved. For the parents of the terminally ill child with cancer, the question becomes what kind of person and what kind of parent will I be if I pursue a particular course of action, rather than how can we eradicate uncertainty through scientific knowledge.

MORAL ORIENTATIONS BASED ON THE PERSPECTIVE OF CARE OR CURE

The perspectives of care and cure also have implications for how moral questions are interpreted and resolved. Consistent with the assumptions of each perspective, the respective moral orientations highlight different features of a situation as morally salient, use different reasoning strategies, emphasize different moral themes, and represent distinct moral concerns that influence how moments of moral ambiguity are interpreted and resolved.[10]

Traditional bioethical theories that emphasize impartiality and rational application of principles and rules are consistent with the cure perspective. For this view, moral choice involves a consideration of moral principles, and reason is the means for adjudicating conflicts among and between competing principles. Within this framework, everyone shares the same rights, duties, and moral obligations and should be governed by the same public norms, rules, and principles.[8,10]

From the perspective of care, moral judgments are viewed as emotional, contextual, and based on the special circumstances of the situation. In other words, the uniqueness of individuals and particular dynamics of their relationships are endorsed as essential components of moral decision-making. Sensitivity to subjective differences is a crucial dimension of the care perspective, whereas the traditional or cure orientation emphasizes objectivity and the application of universal maxims to resolve moral questions. Rules and principles play a secondary role in informing and illuminating moral choice from a care perspective. Principles alone are not determinants of moral activity, although they may have an important role in the moral analysis. Moral responses are, therefore, individualized and guided more by the private norms of friendship, love and care, rather than by abstract rights and principles.[8,9,10]

Classifying certain disciplines, genders, or individuals into an exclusive world view (care or cure) would be a disservice to each discipline and to their individuality. However, various professions have demonstrated a general affinity to a particular perspective that can be useful for examining the decision-making process. Medicine, for example, is most commonly associated with the cure perspective, whereas nursing and family concerns are often associated with the care perspective. But, neither operates in an exclusive domain.

Frequently not only physicians but also other health care providers, as well as patients and families, expect that technology and its attendant hope for cure will come to their aid when they are faced with suspected or obvious disease. Often when the patient is acutely ill the technology is welcomed, especially at first. But, when the technology overshadows what is important to the individual, patients or their families may begin to view the technology as the enemy rather than the ally.

Moreover, physicians may be guided by concerns about family integrity, future quality of life, and the impact of certain decisions on the entire family when they make recommendations about treatment, and it may be families or nurses that indignantly demand that "everything possible" be done to prolong life. In reality, most professionals and family members vacillate between the two perspectives as treatment for an individual child evolves.

The benefit of sensitizing each individual to their prevailing paradigm for decision-making is that it can create an opportunity for a balanced appreciation of the other perspectives when decisions are made. Moreover, it can legitimize allowing all the voices that are represented by various participants to be heard, respected, and taken seriously during the deliberation about the child's best interests.

THE NATURE OF CONFLICTS BETWEEN PROFESSIONALS

The differences in the prevailing perspectives of care and cure have been explored. In the remaining sections of this chapter, the focus will be primarily on the professional conflicts that arise in the care of critically or terminally ill children. Because of the differences in world views, conflicts can occur as a result of differences in values or power, or authority. Often such conflicts result in moral distress or outrage and caregiver suffering.[11] For the purposes of explicating the issues that arise in clinical practice, the following case will be used as a common point of reference.

The Case of Anna: Anna, an ten-month-old infant with perinatally acquired human immunodeficiency virus (HIV), has been hospitalized repeatedly for a variety of HIV-related health problems including opportunistic infections, recurrent fever and sepsis, thrombocytopenia, impaired myocardial function, chronic diarrhea, encephalopathy, failure to thrive and developmental delay. Six weeks ago, she was admitted to the hospital with respiratory distress, poor oxygenation, fever, and failure to thrive. Her respiratory compromise worsened and she was electively intubated and placed on mechanical ventilation. Her liver and spleen were greatly enlarged, myocardial function diminished secondary to cardiomyopathy, fever was recurrent without an identifiable source, and she manifested evidence of encephalopathy. Over the next week she required maximal ventilatory support and oxygen supplementation and was unable to wean from the ventilator. She also experienced pain from muscle aches, mouth sores, candidiasis, hepatosplenomegaly, and frequent painful procedures.

As Anna's condition deteriorated, controversy regarding the goals of her treatment began to emerge among the health care team. Upon her admission to the ICU she was treated aggressively for respiratory failure and multi-system organ failure. A variety of conventional and innovative therapies were instituted. Some members of the team believed that since our understanding of the trajectory of AIDS in children is evolving, it was imperative that she be treated aggressively. Others were becoming increasingly concerned about the level of Anna's pain and the degree of painful intervention that was needed to maintain her life. Despite numerous attempts to provide adequate pain relief, Anna remained undermedicated for her pain. Some team members, particularly the nurses, believed that Anna was dying and that the interventions they were providing were merely prolonging her suffering and were therefore inhumane.

VALUE CONFLICTS

Because of the differences in world views, nurses and physicians may experience value conflicts about the scope of treatment to be provided, and the degree of suffering and pain permissible for critically ill children. Such value conflicts may become apparent because the moral sensitivities of the various participants are focused on different concerns and facts.

According to James Rest, moral sensitivity refers to the individual's ability to recognize that there is a moral problem or conflict.[12] It involves various modes of perception such as empirical observation, empathy, human contact, and intuition. In the broadest sense it means being attuned to the moral dimensions of the situation, that is, being able to recognize what ought to be significant in the context of the particular situation.

Moral sensitivity encompasses various patterns of reflection and modes of exploration. When one's moral sensitivities are guided by objective facts, rules, formal theories, and generalizations that do not depend on particular experiences, the moral dimensions of a case take on certain characteristics. For example, some of the professionals caring for Anna were not convinced that she was in the terminal phase of her disease, in part because scientific knowledge about the trajectory of AIDS in children is still not settled. Their assessment of her condition was focused on the objective data: physiologic indices, laboratory values, and probabilities based on published data and experience. Uncertainty about outcome was a prime motivation for aggressive intervention. They believed that even though her condition was tenuous, it might be reversible and that stopping before they had tried conventional and some innovative therapies would be unjustified.

Others believed that every available therapy ought to be tried to give her a chance to live. From this perspective, a high threshold of burdens could be tolerated to achieve survival. By categorically applying the sanctity of life rule that says life should always be preserved, it was their view that aggressive treatment was indicated. Their perspective was that because life can be sustained, it must be. This principle, for some, had even greater force because Anna was a young child, and so had, potentially, so much life to be saved.

Such an account of the clinical situation may also be focused on the factual or technical dimensions of events, or reflect a procedural concern about meeting minimal standards of conduct for rights and justice. The health care professionals who hold this view may respond to suggestions about limiting treatment by appealing to the quantitative evidence (the "numbers" show progress), institutional rules (you can't limit treatment in cases like this) or invoke the law to support their view (it's against the law to forego treatment). In Anna's case, the law may be used to support continued treatment by interpreting the Federal regulations from the 1984 Child Abuse Prevention and Treatment Act as an imperative for prolonging life. (see Chapter 2.) Legal concerns about discrimination based on a diagnosis of mental or physical handicap could be advanced as a rationale for aggressive intervention.

By contrast, the emotions, intuitions and "gut feelings" can be used as a barometer to locate the salient features or the important dimensions of a situation. Often our emotions signal important aspects of the situation and motivate us to take action.[13] For example, nurses caring for Anna became aware of the moral tensions surrounding her care through their own emotional responses. It was their emotional responses to her suffering that helped them to locate what was at stake in her case. They responded with compassion to her physical and psychosocial suffering as a result of their own anguish about providing treatments that seemed more like torture than care. Their sensitivity to her suffering motivated them to question whether the burdens associated with her treatment were disproportionate in relation to the expected benefits, in effect saying "Why are we doing this?"

Unfortunately, the emotions are often viewed as irrational and disruptive forces, particularly by those guided by the cure perspective. Traditionally, the emotions have been viewed as a distraction that obscures rational judgement.[14] When moral assessments are made, we are advised to arrive at our decisions devoid of emotions by using rational considerations alone. We are advised to step back from our emotions and to make decisions during a "cool hour", instead of in the heat of the moment. For the paradigm of rationality and objectivity, issues that are discussed emotionally are often discounted as illegitimate. Hence, when nurses, who have been sensitized and motivated by their emotions, attempt to raise important issues about treatment, they are often viewed as being overly involved in the situation and, therefore, "unprofessional". Such differences in world views often leave little common ground for discussing the central moral questions openly and constructively.

The collision of such divergent modes of moral sensitivity leads to value conflicts that cannot be resolved quickly or easily. Only if individuals are sensitized to the different moral dimensions of the situation, will they begin to examine the various values that are in conflict. To assess the value conflicts effectively, it is imperative that the individuals have insight into how their own values affect their view of the particular situation. Such clarity of values is often lacking, regardless of how one approaches such dilemmas. Lack of clarity about one's personal and professional values can lead to inconsistent decisions, poorly justified analysis, and moral unrest.

BALANCING BENEFIT AND BURDEN

One of the most common value conflicts in the care of infants and children arises over attempts to balance the benefits and burdens associated with treatment. Nurses in particular experience profound conflicts regarding the burdens associated with treatment interventions. They are often the instruments for carrying out the burdensome interventions that are dictated by the treatment plan. Rarely are their physician colleagues engaged in the round-the-clock interventions that are necessary to sustain life. The ill child's physical characteristics, helplessness, and dependency demand involvement and contact with his or her caregivers in order to survive. Such close proximity allows the nurse to develop an intimate acquaintance with the child and his or her unique responses to the medical and nursing interventions. During periods of extended care, the nurse begins to know the patient in a unique way and becomes greatly invested in his or her well-being. As a result of their relationship with the child and their close proximity to them, many nurses experience profound value conflicts. Not only do nurses have obligations to prolong life, but they are also obliged to diminish pain and suffering and promote a peaceful death. The overriding tension arises between *beneficence* — the duty to do good, and *nonmaleficence* — the duty to avoid harm.

One factor that contributes to this tension is related to differences in professional orientation and moral sensitivity. Each profession has a different set of daily experiences that defines the contours of the information used in making prognostic judgements and in reaching decisions about the efficacy of treatment for a particular patient.[2] For example, nurses may view Anna's response to therapy as an indication that a therapy cannot achieve its intended goal or that the treatment itself is disproportionately burdensome in relation to the expected benefit.[15] Their attention is focused on the physiologic and behavioral responses to therapy. Nurses, for example, are trained to make highly discriminating observations about the children for whom they care. They use technical criteria, behavioral observations, subtle cues, and a cumulative assessment of well-being to inform their judgements about the efficacy of certain interventions and the child's prognosis.[2] Moreover, while technology, drugs, and surgical techniques are highly effective in forestalling death, there are often morbidities including iatrogenic complications that influence the nurse's assessment of benefit and burden. In Anna's case, such a view would likely encompass the whole range of the child's existence: evidence of cumulative physiologic progress, the amount of time spent enduring painful procedures, the level of pain and the effectiveness of interventions to relieve it, whether meaningful interaction is possible and at what frequency, etc. Based on such data, these professionals may believe that the burdens are too great for the small chance that life, meaningful life, may be prolonged.

In contrast, other health care professions may interpret the same responses as an indication that there is a chance that the therapy may achieve its intended goal. Professionals who are guided by a cure perspective are likely to focus on technical criteria such as physical appearance, laboratory data, ventilator settings, and the intensity of care required to achieve the physiologic result.[2] In Anna's case, the physicians or other health care professionals may believe that a 5–10% chance of prolonging life is worth it, despite the burdens that accompany treatment. They would interpret stable or improving physiologic indices as evidence that prolonging life is possible and therefore, beneficial. Such differences in perception of the same situation can result in opposing conclusions about the child's treatment.[2]

When nurses, such as those caring for Anna, have reached their threshold for doubting that their ministrations are promoting the patient's interests, they begin to question the efficacy of the treatment plan. Often these conflicts involve situations in which the goals of treatment are unclear or in conflict. In Anna's case, the goals of the medical team were to correct her physiologic impairments and restore her to her previous state of health. In contrast, the nursing goal was to minimize pain and suffering and to promote a peaceful death. Without unity and clarity of goals to guide decision making, inconsistent and incongruent decisions are likely to be made. Moreover, the integrity, self-esteem, and morale of the professionals is often sacrificed for the sake of continued treatment.

Nurses and other health care professionals may also experience conflicts which arise when their responsibility to promote the patient's well-being clash with the perspective of the family. Consider Anna's case again. Perhaps it might not be the physician, but rather the family who requests that "everything" be done to sustain life. As the case unfolds, Anna's condition continues to deteriorate and she becomes more physiologically unstable, requiring maximal ventilatory and pharmacologic support. The physicians now agree that they have reached their maximal therapeutic level, that her condition is no longer reversible and that she is dying. But, when they suggest to Anna's mother that she should not be resuscitated if she should arrest and that treatment should not be escalated, she refuses the idea of a do-not-resuscitate (DNR) order and again demands that everything be done to sustain her daughter's life. In this situation, nurses and physicians may be forced to provide care that is contrary to their moral values and professional obligations. They may believe that to honor the mother's request to continue aggressive treatment compromises their ability to provide humane treatment and undermines their professional integrity.

Such situations raise important questions about how such conflicts ought to be resolved and by whom. Families, for example, may be socialized into the medical model by taking cues from health care providers about what information is pertinent about the child's condition. They begin to focus on laboratory values and vital signs rather than on a holistic picture of their child's condition. Additionally, they may be receiving incongruent messages about their child's condition from various health care team members or they may not be processing information at the same rate or in the same manner as the professionals who are providing care and giving feedback about the child's condition.[16] The health care professionals themselves may also be struggling to define a morally defensible plan of care for Anna as they attempt to balance their competing obligations to the patient, family, and themselves. (For further examination of this issue, see Chapter 9, The Limits of the Physician's Duty to Treat.)

CAUSING PAIN AND SUFFERING

Another potential value conflict involves an additional dimension of balancing benefit and harms, that is, determining what is "appropriate" relief of pain and suffering. The issue of adequate pain management has become an ethical issue of significant proportions, particularly when children are involved.[17] Moreover, the direct infliction of painful procedures particularly those associated with marginally effective treatments causes moral conflicts for caregivers, particularly nurses.[18] In one study, NICU nurses identified issues related to pain, suffering and humane treatment of infants as a principal source of moral conflict in their practice.[19]

Nurses in particular are sensitive to their role in the infliction of pain and suffering on infants and children. Nurses are required to provide safe, effective treatment and to promote comfort. Nurses routinely carry out painful and invasive procedures that are required by the treatment of critically and terminally ill children. They are attuned to the nuances of the child's responses to treatments, which informs their interpretation of such interventions as beneficial or harmful. It is often their sustained participation in these activities and their close proximity to the child that allows for their continued assessment of whether such interventions are humane.

The nurses caring for Anna recognized the pain and suffering associated with her treatment. They were continually reminded of the burden of her treatment by their observations of her vital signs, behavior, level of awareness and interaction, and physical appearance. After suctioning, for example, Anna would become agitated, diaphoretic, and inconsolable for 30 to 45 minutes. Based on their assessment of her condition as end-stage, their primary goal became comfort. They advocated a variety of measures to achieve pain relief and comfort including pharmacologic and non-pharmacologic measures. Since they did not believe that Anna could be restored to her previous state, they were willing to accept some compromise in their ability to assess her condition in order to achieve adequate pain relief. Moreover, because she was dying, they believed that the provision of adequate analgesia was indicated even if it secondarily foreshortened her life. Their goals, however, were in opposition to the goals of the medical team.

The medical team was concerned about Anna's comfort but their primary concern was discovering the optimal combination of interventions to sustain her life. They were willing to institute only those measures that would not interfere with their ability to monitor the effects of their interventions. They were, for example, unwilling to administer doses of analgesia that were necessary to alleviate her pain because they believed that to do so could impair their ability to accurately assess her neurologic status or cause physiologic instability. Because their goal was to correct the underlying problem, continued neurologic competence was a key component of their determination of beneficial treatment. Such disparities in values and world views produced moral conflicts over the proper balance between benefitting the patient and causing harm. (For further discussion of this issue, see Chapter 11, "Pain, Hurt and Harm: The Ethical Issue of Pediatric Pain Control".)

UNEQUAL POWER OR AUTHORITY

When conflict occurs in cases like Anna's, it is often a result of actual or perceived inequality in power or authority. Traditionally, relationships in health care settings are hierarchical; power comes from achieving power over others or taking power away from others. Power is viewed as of limited quantities.[20] The power paradigm is controlling, authoritarian, competitive, and divisive. The hierarchy of the medical system promotes inequality in power and authority among various health care team members and families. Physicians have traditionally been in charge of treatment decisions with patients, families and other professionals playing a subordinate role. Normally physicians make treatment decisions; other professionals do not.

Yet it is the nurse who spends countless, intimate hours with patients and their families and who witnesses the consequences of the decisions of others. Although nurses are regularly called upon to implement plans they may view as burdensome, their input into decision-making may not be sought or may be disregarded. When nurses, for example, perceive that they have no control over their own practice or have no input into the treatment plan, both their moral agency and their professional integrity are threatened. Their values become suppressed by following rules or policies that limit or discount the legitimate role of the nurse in the decision-making process.[21] Often when this disparity in power is coupled with divergent views of the treatment plan, conflict escalates.

The tensions produced by such disparities in perceptions of power and authority can distract caregivers from focusing on what is best for the patient. It may cause nurses, such as those caring for Anna, to resort to passive–aggressive communication styles in which they "disguise opinions as suggestions and circumvent conflict by withholding information or contributions that may improve patient care."[22] Similarly, physicians may invoke their authority as the "captain of the ship" to avoid conflict and confrontation. They may, for example, resist the nurses' "suggestions" about ways to manage Anna's pain and suffering; or they may ignore a request for a patient care conference to discuss her plan of care. Such tactics may be effective in the short term, but ultimately each profession suffers because the interprofessional conflicts become internalized and incarcerated rather than being openly dealt with. In the end, patient care is compromised.

PROFESSIONAL CONFLICTS AND MORAL DISTRESS

Professional conflicts that are not satisfactorily resolved can result in moral distress. Moral distress occurs when nurses or other health professionals are unable to translate their moral choices into moral action.[23] Acting in a manner that goes against personal or professional values is an attack on the individual's integrity or authenticity. When professionals cannot live up to their personal values by acting in an ethical manner, they experience moral distress. In a recent study by Solomon *et al.*, 50% of the nearly 760 nursing respondents reported that they had acted against their consciences in providing care to the terminally ill. Of the physician respondents in the same study, 32–34% of attending physicians and 70% of house officers reported acting against their consciences. In both groups, those who reported acting against their conscience were more likely to report concerns about over-treatment, rather than concerns about under-treatment.[24]

The magnitude of moral distress that may be occurring in our clinical settings on a daily basis is unknown but it is suspected to be quite common, particularly among nurses and physicians in training. If their distress is unrelieved, the individual's self-worth is jeopardized, personal and professional relationships may be affected, and psychological changes, behavioral manifestations, and physical symptoms may occur. Ultimately, as with all unresolved inter-professional conflicts, the quality of patient care suffers.[25]

STRATEGIES FOR BLENDING CARE AND CURE

At different times and under varying circumstances, individual practitioners, patients, and families may vacillate between the perspectives of cure and care. In order for all the participants in the illness experience to maintain their integrity, there must be some effort to identify, respect and reconcile their views of morality and science. One important dimension of this process is agreeing on a strategy for framing the issues.

Clearly a balance between the cure and care perspectives must be sought. Herein lies the challenge for professionals of all disciplines. All participants must be aware of their own prevailing values and patterns of decision-making before they will be able to recognize and appreciate the viewpoints of others. A culture must be fostered among all disciplines that promotes acknowledging and respecting diversity, providing opportunities for divergent views to be heard and considered, and striving for treatment plans that everyone can live with. When this is not possible, creating the kind of practice environment where individual practitioners can remove themselves from morally objectionable situations without fear of ostracism, reprisal or disrespectful treatment must be encouraged.

True collaboration must occur for the perspectives of care and cure to be blended into a "synergistic alliance" that maximizes the contributions of each participant.[25] Non-hierarchical relationships that are interdependent and based on mutual respect and trust must be developed. Such a model of relationships promotes the sharing of responsibility and accountability by each participant in the moral struggle. The social and political climate of individual units and institutions, and of the members who practice therein must be altered significantly to allow for the previously silenced perspectives represented by concerns for care to become audible. An essential ingredient in the collaborative relationship is honest, open, and respectful dialogue that supports synergy rather than antagonism between the various perspectives. Moreover, such relationships must be nurtured and supported over time. Trust and mutual respect can only thrive when constant groups of providers work together over time.[25]

Authentic collaboration is built on a foundation of empowerment rather than a hierarchical power relationship. "Empowerment implies the creation of a new reality which differs from the current and pervasive power paradigm."[26] The empowered individual is willing and eager to assist others in realizing their full potential by supporting, encouraging, challenging and coaching them in their efforts. This requires an environment which supports the discovery and mastery of personal power and cultivates growth by providing support, commitment of time and energy, and the provision of safety nets for professionals.[26]

Moreover, it is essential to create mechanisms for shared governance that provide opportunities for active participation for all in the identification and resolution of patient care issues, and that clearly define the scope of responsibility and accountability of each profession.

A congruent philosophy about patient care, family involvement in decision-making, and professional relationships is also a key ingredient in creating an ethical practice environment. Such a philosophy must be patient/family-centered, based on humanistic values, and be guided toward healing. As Pellegrino and Thomasma have argued, healing ought to be the goal of our clinical endeavors. They assert that healing encompasses much more than curing and incorporates physiologic, psychologic, social and spiritual dimensions. "To heal is to make whole or sound, to help a person reconvene the powers of the self and return, as far as possible, to his conception of a normal life."[27]

Inherent in an ethical practice environment are opportunities for interdisciplinary discourse, analysis, and education. For example, monthly interdisciplinary ethics rounds, regular educational opportunities for ethics education, the inclusion of ethics content in orientation programs, and forums for case analysis can contribute to meaningful dialogue and discussion. The mark of the success of such endeavors is the establishment of a climate of openness, trust, and support. Participants must become adept at clarifying their own values and helping others to do the same. Divergent viewpoints must be heard and respected and differences in opinion handled without malice or reprisal.

When conflicts emerge, supportive mechanisms for dispute resolution are essential. This includes having an interdisciplinary ethics committee or consultation service available for timely activation by all members of the health care team, patients, and families. The deliberations of the committee must be balanced and ethically defensible. Moreover, the establishment of written institutional policies governing foregoing treatment, resuscitation, artificially provided hydration and nutrition, informed consent, innovative practices, research, the scope of professional responsibility, and guidelines for judicial intervention provide prudent safeguards.

Professionals can only thrive in supportive environments. Employee assistance programs, mental health services, support groups, and professional development opportunities will contribute to the well-being of professionals. Such services must be easily accessible and viewed as beneficial by caregivers.

CONCLUSION

The challenges of providing care to critically and terminally ill children and their families are daunting. One essential step toward satisfactory resolution of the conflicts that arise in their treatment is to blend the world views represented by care and cure. Attention to such issues will ultimately result in improved outcomes for patients and families and enhanced satisfaction for all professionals. Such efforts can contribute substantially to the development of a truly ethical practice environment that preserves the integrity of all participants and fosters reasoned deliberations and morally defensible outcomes.

References

1. Visintainer, M. (1986). The nature of knowledge and theory in nursing. *IMAGE: The Journal of Nursing Scholarship*, **18**:32–38.
2. Anspach, R. (1987). Prognostic conflict in life and death decisions: The organization as an ecology of knowledge. *Journal of Health and Social Behavior*, **28**:215–231.
3. Fischer, A. and Stevenson, D. (1987). The consequences of uncertainty: An empirical approach to medical decision-making in neonatal intensive care. *JAMA*, **258**:1929–1931.
4. Able-Boone, H., Dokecki, P. and Smith, S. (1989). Parent and health care provider communication and decision-making in the intensive care nursery. *Children's Health Care*, **18**:133–141.
5. Bogdan, R., Brown, M. and Foster, S. (1982). Be honest but not cruel: Staff/parent communication on neonatal unit. *Human Organization*, **41**:6–16.
6. Engelhardt, H. T. (1986). *The Foundations of Bioethics* pp. 157–97, New York: Oxford University Press.
7. Bursztajin, H. J., Feinbloom, F. I., Hamm, R. M. and Brodsky, A. (1990). *Medical Choices, Medical Chances* New York: Routledge.
8. Cooper, M. C. (1991). Principle-oriented ethics and the ethic of care: A creative tension. *Advances in Nursing Science*, **14(2)**:22–31.
9. Gilligan, C. (1982). *In a Different Voice: Psychological Theory and Women's Development* pp. 5–23, Cambridge, Mass.: Harvard University Press.
10. Carse, A. (1991). The voice of care: Implications for bioethical education. *J. Med. Philos.*, **16**:5–28.
11. Rushton, C. H. (1992). Caregiver suffering in critical care nursing. *Heart & Lung*, **21(3)**:303–6.
12. Rest, J. (1986). An overview of the psychology of morality. *Moral Development: Advances in Research and Theory* pp. 1–27, New York: Praeger.
13. Hinman, L. (1985). Emotion, morality and understanding. In: C. G. Harding (ed) *Moral Dilemmas* p. 66, Chicago: Precedent Publishing.
14. Callahan, S. (1988). The role of emotion in ethical decision-making. *The Hastings Center Report*, **18**:9–14.
15. Nelson, L. J. and Nelson, R. M. (1992). Ethics and the provision of futile, harmful or burdensome treatment to children. *Critical Care Medicine*, **20**:427–433.
16. King, N. P. (1992). Transparency in neonatal intensive care. *Hastings Center Report*, **22(2)**:18–25.
17. Franck, L. S. (1992). The influence of sociopolitical, scientific, and technologic forces on the study and treatment of neonatal pain. *Advances in Nursing Science*, **15**:11–20.
18. Penticuff, J. H. (1992). The impact of the Child Abuse Amendments on nursing staff and their care of handicapped newborns. In: *Compelled Compassion: Government Intervention in the Treatment of Critically Ill Newborns* A. L. Caplan, R. H. Blank, J. C. Merrick (eds) Totowa, N. J.: Humana Press pp. 267–282.
19. Miya, P. A., Boardman, K. K., Harr, K. L. and Keene, A. (1991). Ethical issues described by neonatal nurses. *Journal of Clinical Ethics*, **2**:253–257.
20. Starhawk, J. (1982). *Dreaming the Dark: Magic, Sex and Politics* Boston: Beacon Press.
21. Reich, W. T. (1991). Caring as extraordinary means. *Second Opinion*, **17**:46–56.
22. Allen, M. L., Jackson, D. and Youngner, S. (1980). Closing the communication gap between physicians and nurses in the intensive care setting. *Heart & Lung*, **9(5)**:836–840.

23. Wilkinson, J. M. (1987/88). Moral distress in nursing practice: Experience and effect. *Nursing Forum*, **23**:16–29.
24. Soloman, M. Z., O'Donnell, L., Jennings, B., Guilfoy, V., Wolfe, S., Nolan, K., *et al.,* (1993). Desicions near the end of life: Professional views on life-sustaining treatments. *Am. J. Public Health*, **83(1)**:14–23.
25. Pike, A. (1991). Moral outrage and moral discourse in nurse-physician collaboration. *J. Prof. Nurs.*, **7(6)**:351–363.
26. Richmond, T. (1992). Empowering onself through others. Unpublished manuscript p. 1.
27. Pellegrino, E. D. and Thomasma, D. C. (1988). *For the Patient's Good* p. 10 New York: Oxford University Press.

11 Pain, Hurt, and Harm: The Ethical Issue of Pediatric Pain Control*

Robert C. Cassidy[1] and Gary A. Walco[2]

[1]Schneider Children's Hospital, Long Island Jewish Medical Center and
[2]Tomorrow's Children's Institute, H.ackensack Medical Center

Is it ethical to allow children to suffer more than they have to? The answer to this question seems obvious. Yet, for many years this issue has been focal in the protracted debate over pain control. It has long been recognized that patients receive less relief from pain than they should.[1,2] Ferrel and Rhiner[3] used World Health Organization data on cancer pain to reach the following conclusions: Pain could be relieved effectively for 90% of patients but, pain was relieved effectively for only 20% of patients. As the editor of the *New England Journal of Medicine* declares:

> Few things a doctor does are more important than relieving pain. Yet the treatment of severe pain in hospitalized patients is regularly and systematically inadequate.[4]

Most pertinent for our pediatric concerns, and perhaps most surprising to our humane sense, clinical surveys reveal that the general tendency toward under medication of pain is even more pronounced in children. A review of studies on post-operative pain indicated huge disparities in the amount of analgesia ordered for adults versus children.[5] An investigation from the mid 1970's, for example, showed that 25 children between the ages of 4 and 8 years who had undergone major surgical procedures (amputations, nephrectomies, atrial septal defects), had received only 24 doses of analgesic medication. By contrast, 18 adult surgical patients in the same institution undergoing similar procedures received 671 doses of analgesic.[6] More recent findings show no significant improvement. A 1991 study at a major Boston teaching hospital found that while adults routinely received local anesthesia for lumbar puncture, there was no evidence that any of 252 children received any analgesic care.[7]

Although it is clear that interest in pediatric pain control has blossomed over the past decade, a recurrent theme in a recent "state of the art" text[8] is still the consistent incongruity between what is available technologically and what is practiced clinically. Confronted by this disparity, we must deal with an urgent ethical question: Is the apparent undertreatment of pain in children ethically justifiable? If the answer to this question is "No!", then the ethical duty of all pediatric caregivers must be to increase pain relief for children.

*An earlier version of this chapter appeared as "Pain, Hurt, and Harm: The Ethics of Pain Control in Infants and Children" in the *New England Journal of Medicine*, 1994, **331**:541–544.

However, the answer is not so obvious, since pain is not always an unqualified evil, and pain relief interventions are not always of unqualified benefit. After all, the determinative principle of responsible medical care is not "Do No *Hurt*." It is "Do No *Harm*." The difference is that the most appropriate medical treatment often entails hurting a patient (certain invasive diagnostic procedures, for example). Harm only occurs when either the amount of hurt is greater than the amount of benefit, or when the amount of hurt is greater than necessary to achieve the intended benefit.

Therefore, the basic ethical challenge to caregivers is this: Since pain seems on the face of it harmful for patients, and caregivers are categorically committed to preventing harm to their patients. How do you justify not using all available means of pain relief?

Possible justifications can be divided into three basic types: (a) a *Revisionist* Justification: The pain is not that bad; (b) a *Comparative* Justification: The pain is not the worst; and (c) a *Pragmatic* Justification: The pain may produce something better. The nature and limitations of these three licenses for undertreatment of pain need to be explored in more detail.

THE REVISIONIST JUSTIFICATION

> Years ago the daughter of one of us fell and skinned her knee. The good father rushed to comfort her; but when his efforts failed, he said, "Come on now, dear. It doesn't hurt *that* much." To which she responded, "It doesn't hurt *you* that much, Daddy."

Due to the nature of the symptoms and the emotional responses they may evoke, pain treatment traditionally has depended more on subjective rather than objective judgements by caregivers. Fundamentally, pain is a private experience to which no other person can gain direct access. Thus, based on factors such as knowledge of the specific pathophysiology and behavioral observations of the child, caregivers make some judgement about the individual's pain experience.[9] The fact that pain is undertreated in children implies, therefore, that the relationships among pain, the severity of the pathophysiology, and pain behavior are not direct, and/or that caregivers are not objective behavioral observers. The problem becomes even more complicated because caregivers' judgements regarding pain assessment and intervention are subject to their own deep-seated standards and views about human behavior.[10]

When it comes to pain, we often minimize the validity of children's self-reports. Rather, we assess the "evidence" presented by the child, weighing the quantity and quality of the behavior against our sense of the "correct" or "appropriate" amount of pain.[11] Further, the respect for parental license to speak and act for their children reinforces this disenfranchising of the child's own cries. We turn to parents (appropriately at some developmental levels) to get a pain history, to find out what's "really" happening. Often, we also get a pain interpretation which expresses a character assessment (e.g., "She has always been a fussy child," or "He is usually quite brave."). The child's pain experience gets filtered and edited into a revisionist judgement which typically minimizes the child's pain. This in turn results in minimizing the amount of analgesia judged "necessary."

Why is the revisionist perspective utilized to justify less relief? First, there is the mistaken notion that there is a "correct" amount of pain. The error results from the myth that there is (or should be) a uniform response for a given pathophysiologic condition or pain stimulus. Despite extensive studies of the individuation of pain responses in children, going back to the seminal work of Petrie in the 1960's, some caregivers still insist on ignoring the individual child and treating their own prejudged "appropriate" child.[12–14]

Recent empirical studies support these points. Consider, for example, the relationship between relatively objective measures of nociceptive stimulation (pathophysiology) and estimates of pain intensity. Theoretically, if physicians' ratings of patients' pain rely heavily on knowledge of the disease process with minimal subjective bias, that correlation should be fairly high. However, in a study of the relationship between heat in joints affected by juvenile rheumatoid arthritis and visual analogue scale ratings of patients' pain intensity by physicians, that correlation was $r = .57$, indicating that 67 percent of the variance in patients' pain experience was unaccounted for.[15]

The paternalistic sense that we adults know better than the child how bad it is, may be reinforced by other adult concerns. For example, our fear that children will fake or exaggerate suffering to obtain some secondary gain may cause us to disparage their pain accounts in order to protect our need to feel in control.[11] Our needs may also lead us to downplay a child's suffering in order to anesthetize ourselves to our own otherwise unbearable anguish. As pediatric pain is often extremely difficult to treat, we may be inclined to blame the child for protesting too much in order to alleviate the burden of our not relieving enough.[16]

The feelings of caregivers (both professional and familial) and their resulting judgements also may be insulated by ignorance about the nature of pediatric pain. As technology has advanced, commonly held myths about children's pain experiences have been discredited. First was the belief that very young infants, in particular, did not have the neurological capacity to experience pain. More sophisticated means of assessing neuroanatomical development[17], as well as more disciplined means of measuring behavioral responses, such as spectrographic analysis of infant cries[18] and physiologic responses, specifically sympathetic nervous system arousal[19], have demonstrated that even very young infants experience painful stimuli. Most impressive, however, are the data from Anand and colleagues in which it has been shown that premature infants undergoing operations with minimal anesthesia, which was standard practice, had significantly higher stress responses (measured by hormonal and metabolic indices) and significantly higher complication and mortality rates post-operatively.[20,21]

The strongest argument against the myth that children do not feel pain comes from the consensus of the current neuroanatomic data. Pain pathways and cortical and subcortical centers necessary for pain perception are well developed late in gestation, and neurological systems known to be associated with pain transmission and modulation are also intact and functional.[17]

A related misunderstanding was the belief that, even if very young children did experience pain, they had no enduring memory of the experience. From this (ungrounded) impression, some concluded that since children's pain was merely momentary, it was not significant. However, recent studies have yielded substantive evidence that pain and the trauma associated with painful experience produce enduring memory as manifested in behavioral changes, such as disturbances of feeding, sleeping, and state control after acute pain experiences.[22] Preliminary data also suggest that early pain experiences have permanent effects on the development of pain-receptive neural pathways, which may in turn produce lasting effects on the individual's later pain experiences.[23]

Another discredited belief is that children's pain could not be measured. A review of the literature in this area is well beyond the scope of this article. Briefly, however, pain in children may be assessed through physiologic indicators, systematic observation of pain behavior, and the self-report of the child.[24] In clinical settings, the latter two are most prevalent. A number of studies have shown the reliability, validity, and clinical utility of structured behavioral ratings to measure discrete aspects of children's pain and distress associated with invasive procedures[25–27] and post-operative pain.[28]

McGrath[24] provides a detailed review of methods available for measuring various aspects of self-reported pain in children. The key psychometric properties have been addressed and the consensus in the field is that children from about 5 years of age and up are very reliable reporters of their own pain experience. Therefore, if there are discrepancies between parent, physician, and child reports of a child's pain, it usually makes the most sense to defer to the child's perspective.[29] Since the data document the reliability of children's reports, informed practitioners should no longer assume that anybody else knows better than the child what he or she is really experiencing.

In order to justify minimizing pain interventions on revisionist grounds, one must claim to know the other person's internal state better than that person knows himself or herself. Based on the aforementioned data, as well as human considerations and common sense, this position is no longer defensible. Children feel pain and are able to communicate that response in a number of ways. The caregiver's job is to utilize the available strategies in order to more sensitively observe, more objectively assess, and more responsively treat the child's condition. Denying relief proportionate to expressed need must be judged an unjustified harm, unless such deliberate deprivation serves some substantially greater good.

THE COMPARATIVE JUSTIFICATION

Even if we were to agree that pain in and of itself is real and bad, we still would have to decide how bad it is for the child by comparing it to the relevant alternatives. Only then would we know how to act. In other words, even if we accept children's self-reported pain as a reality, we would still have to weigh the pluses and minuses of unrelieved pain against those of pain relief. A responsible and responsive assessment of all the consequences of the options might lead to a conclusion that, all things considered, the harm of unrelieved pain may be less severe than the harm of pain relief.

This is the Comparative Justification for choosing pain as the lesser evil. Three aspects of analgesic relief have usually been considered when the judgement is that pain is the lesser evil: (1) the method of administration, (2) the danger of side effects, and (3) the long-term consequences of use, such as addiction. Once again, recent data indicate that many of the long-held concerns about these issues are questionable.

Focusing first on routes of administration of analgesics, traditionally the management of moderate to severe acute pain in children employed needles for the parenteral administration of narcotics. Especially in young children, the fear (inordinate, perhaps, but nevertheless real) of the needle often produced painfully real discomfort and distress. The anxiety and resultant agitation could short-circuit cooperation and compromise treatment. In some circumstances the solution could be worse than the problem, and potent analgesics were withheld in order to avoid painful injections.

However, we are now able to circumvent the problem through more creative routes of administration. For example, vaso-occlusive pain in sickle cell disease may be managed through the same intravenous lines for hydration, thereby obviating the need for additional injections. Post-operative pain may be managed in a similar fashion, as most children coming out of surgery have an intravenous line in place. Patient controlled analgesia may also be utilized. In addition, anesthesiologists may chose to administer epidural medications during the post-operative period which involve minimal discomfort for the patient, yet provide excellent analgesia.

A second major concern is the potential for problematic side effects of some analgesic medications. Chief on the list is respiratory depression associated with narcotics, apparently due to reductions in brain stem respiratory center sensitivity to hypercarbia and hypoxia.[30] While this fact is not disputed, the relevant issues to be considered are: (1) What is the incidence of respiratory depression secondary to narcotic administration in small children? (2) Is the risk of respiratory problems greater in children than in adults? (3) Do the side effects associated with narcotics, such as respiratory depression, pose a serious and irreversible threat?

These issues were reviewed in detail by McCafferty and Wong.[31] They concluded that the risk of narcotic induced respiratory depression in adults is about 0.09%.[32] The rates of such difficulties in children were shown to be 0%[33] in one study and approximately 1.3% in another.[34] It should also be noted that among over 600 patients in the latter study, only one required naloxone as opposed to a simple dose reduction to correct the problem. Thus, there are no data to support the notion that children are more susceptible to this problem than are adults. By following appropriate dosing guidelines and adequately monitoring patients, respiratory depression is likely to be prevented. If problematic side effects do occur, an opioid antagonist such as naloxone is a quick and effective way to reverse all narcotic effects.[35]

Finally, the fear of addiction creates substantial concerns about analgesic administration. Survey data indicate that 39% of physicians were somewhat or significantly concerned about the risk of addiction resulting from narcotic analgesic usage in young patients.[36] Such physicians' concerns may be strongly reinforced by parents' anxious objections to giving narcotics to their children.[10]

Once again, however, the data do not support these fears. It is essential to differentiate between physical dependence (a physiologic response as tolerance builds with repeated administration of narcotics) and addiction (a psychological dependence on the drug). It is noteworthy that narcotic addiction is quite rare among adults treated for disease-related pain and appears to be dependent on factors beyond narcotic administration.[37] Studies among pediatric patients treated for pain associated with sickle cell disease[38,39] and post-operative recovery[34] have demonstrated virtually no risk of addiction associated with narcotic administration. Finally, there are no known aspects of childhood physiology or psychology that would make children more vulnerable to addiction than adults.

For the advocates of "adequate" pain relief, such concerns are an inordinate expression of caregivers' unfounded fears. These anxieties exaggerate the risks of analgesic induced addiction, and lead one to minimize the harms of untreated pain. As Angell declares:

> I can't think of any other area in medicine in which such an extravagant concern for side effects so drastically limits treatment. We are used to a closer balance between risks and benefits.[40]

In all fairness, however, while the grounds for fearing post-analgesic addiction are anecdotal at best, Schechter and Allen[36] point out that there are no specific studies on addiction in children who received narcotics for pain. As reports on the lack of addiction to narcotics administered for pain are often not systematic, well-controlled studies of this issue are needed. Based on the present data, however, it is reasonable to conclude that if analgesics are administered properly, the risk of addiction poses a minimal threat.

We must not permit the fear of a hypothetical side-effect to deafen us to the all-too-real cries for help of children in pain. Any comparative justification for withholding pain relief must be rigorously judged by a disciplined assessment of risks and benefits grounded on empirical data. Speculation and undocumented lore are not professionally acceptable.

THE PRAGMATIC JUSTIFICATION

The Pragmatic Justification authorizes using some means which in-and-of themselves are bad, if the end they serve is good. Its classic formulation is, "The End justifies the Means."

For caregivers, pain is often viewed as a means to an end. Pain is not judged to be good or bad in and of itself, but rather by how it affects the goals of therapy (e.g., cure of disease, prevention of death, improvement of function). For clinicians, suffering may be ethically acceptable if it is therapeutically beneficial.

However, no end justifies any means. Justification requires proportionality. There must be a positive proportionality between the value of the end and the burdens of the means. Treatment is a package deal and our ethical duty is to design the package with the greatest possible benefit and the least possible suffering. Therefore, a Pragmatic Justification is only permissible after we have carefully tested both the Means and the Ends involved in each individual case.

Morality of Means Test

For the end to justify the means, the end must be a substantial and realizable good; and the means used to achieve that good must be reasonably expected to prove effective. Thus, in order to use pain as a therapeutic instrument, a pragmatic "Morality of Means" test must be passed. This test has three component challenges:

(1) *Is the pain useful?* We must be able to affirm that there is a reasonable probability that using the pain will really achieve the end that is sought.

(2) *Is the pain necessary?* Using pain is only justified when there is no other less noxious means available. Pain must be the instrument of last resort.

(3) *Is the pain the least possible?* We must do all we can to assure that only the minimal amount of pain remains. Since the price of the therapeutic gain is paid by the suffering of a child, we must be exquisitely economical.

Morality of Ends Test

In addition to passing the morality of means test, pragmatic justification requires a "Morality of Ends" test. Two major ends or purposes are usually invoked by those who justify pain on pragmatic grounds: Therapeutic Guidance and Character Development. For the Therapeutic Guidance purpose, pain may be viewed as useful to determine the nature and extent of an illness. For example, pain responses observed while palpating a child's abdomen may serve as an important means of diagnosing an ailment. Similarly, pain may be an important indication of the lack of efficacy of a treatment or of the limits of treatment, such as discomfort experienced during physical rehabilitation after orthopedic surgery. In such circumstances, relieving pain might cloud the physician's judgement and, thereby, actually harm the patient. One must weigh the benefits of immediate relief against the benefits of long-term cure or recovery.

The second end used to justify the means of pain, Character Development, is much more ethically dubious. In its most trite form, "No pain, no gain!", it is more appropriate (if at all) in the locker room than in the patient's room. This moralistic theory champions certain character traits such as courage, self-discipline, independence and self-sacrifice. Its variations range from a Spartan military model to a Puritanical religious model in which pain is thought to teach, temper, and test these virtues. Both parents and caregivers may praise children for being "brave" and "grown-up", thereby minimizing the power of pain, and ignoring the child's internal distress. Conversely, the child who expresses pain and cries for help is chided as a disappointment, a weakling, or, that most demeaning pejorative, as "acting like a baby".

Although in some settings promoting such heroic virtues may be ethically defensible, in a medical context they become extremely questionable. Imposing the additional burden of character development on a child already encumbered by sickness and suffering reflects a lack of compassion and may be therapeutically harmful. When eradication of pain is not technologically feasible (such as pain associated with chronic illness), strengthening the child's capacity to cope with the inescapable is beneficial to the child and is justifiable. However, to deliberately withhold available analgesics in order to teach a moral lesson denies respect for the significance of the child's present life and concern for his or her real suffering.

SUMMARY

In conclusion, for many years there was a great deal we did not understand about the assessment and management of pain in children. Without a substantial knowledge base, practitioners were left to rely on their own subjective judgements. These were fraught with inconsistencies and personal biases, and typically led to under treatment of pain. Now we know that the old "myths" have been refuted by solid research data.[6,8] Therefore, as is the case in all areas of medicine, it is incumbent on scientific practitioners to provide care in a manner consistent with the technological growth of the field. Increasingly, guidelines for the assessment and treatment of pediatric pain are being published to educate and direct the practice of pediatric caregivers,[41–44] and these must be implemented in everyday practice. Reliance on outmoded attitudes, no matter how pervasive, and personal biases, no matter how sincere, is irrational and harmful. Both scientific and ethical standards demand that undertreatment of pain be rejected as substandard pediatric practice.

References

1. Marks R. M., Sachar E. J. (1973). Undertreatment of medical patients with narcotic analgesics. *Ann. Int. Med.*, **78**:173–81.
2. World Health Organization (1990). Cancer pain relief and palliative care. Geneva: WHO.
3. Ferrell B. R., Rhiner M. (1991). High-tech comfort: Ethical issues in cancer pain management for the 1990's. *J. Clin. Ethics*, **2**:108–15.
4. Angell, M. (1982). The quality of mercy. *NEJM*, 306:98.
5. Schechter N. L., Allen D. A., Hanson K. (1986). Status of pediatric pain control: A comparison of hospital analgesic usage in children and adults. *Pediatrics*, **77**:11–5.
6. Schechter N. L. (1989). The undertreatment of pain in children: An overview. *Pediatr. Clin. North Am.*, **36**:781–94.
7. Bauchner H. (1991). Procedures, pain and parents. *Pediatrics*, **87**:563–65.
8. Schechter N. L., Berde C. B., Yaster M., eds. (1993). *Pain in infants, children, and adolescents*. Baltimore: Williams & Wilkins.
9. Walco, G. A., Dampier C. D. (1990). Pain in children and adolescents with sickle cell disease: A descriptive study. *J. Pediatr. Psychol.*, **15**:643–58.
10. Nolan K. (1993). Ethical issues in pediatric pain management. In: Schechter N. L., Berde C. B., Yeaster M., eds. *Pain in infants, children, and adolescents*. Baltimore: Williams & Wilkins, 123–32.
11. Hammond D. (1979). Unnecessary suffering: Pain and the doctor-patient relationship. *Perspect Bio. Med.* **23**:152–160.
12. Petrie A. (1967). *Individuality in pain and suffering*. Chicago: University of Chicago Press.
13. Mechanic D. (1980). The experience and reporting of common physical complaints. *J. Health Soc. Behav.*, **21**:146–55.
14. Grunau R., Craig K. D. (1987). *Pain* expression in neonates. *Pain*, **28**:395–410.
15. Ilowite N. T., Walco G. A., Pochaczevsky R. (1992). Pain assessment in juvenile rheumatoid arthritis: relation between pain intensity and degree of joint inflammation. *Ann. Rheum Dis.*, **51**:343–6.
16. McGrath P. J., Craig K. D. (1989). Developmental and psychological factors in children's pain. *Pediatr. Clin. North Am.*, **36**:823–35.
17. Anand K. J. S., Hickey P. R. (1987). Pain in the fetus and neonate. *N. Engl. J. Med.*, **317**:1321–9.
18. Levine J. D., Gordon N. C. (1982). Pain in prelingual children and its evaluation by pain-induced vocalization. *Pain*, **14**:85–93.
19. Williamson P. S., Williamson M. L. (1983). Physiological stress reduction by a local anesthetic during newborn circumcision. *Pediatrics*, **71**:36–40.
20. Anand K. J. S., Sippell W. G., Aynsley-Green A. (1987). Randomized trial of fentanyl anesthesia in preterm babies undergoing surgery: effects on stress response. *Lancet*, **1**:243–8.

21. Anand K. J. S., Carr D. B., Kickey P. R. (1987). Randomized trial of fentanyl anesthesia in preterm babies undergoing surgery: hormonal and hemodynamic stress response. *Anesthesiology*, **67**:A502.
22. Marshall R. E., Stratton W. C., Moore J. A., *et al.*, Circumcision. I. Effects upon newborn behavior. *Infant Behav. Devel.*, **180**:3:1–14.
23. Fitzgerald M., Anand K. J. S. (1993). Developmental neuroanatomy and neurophysiology of pain. In: Schechter N. L., Berde C. B., Yaster, M., eds. *Pain in infants, children, and adolescents*. Baltimore: Williams & Wilkins, 11–31.
24. McGrath P. A. (1987). An assessment of children's pain: a review of behavioral, physiological and direct scaling techniques. *Pain*, **31**:147–176.
25. Jay S. M., Ozolins M., Elliot C. H., Caldwell S. (1983). Assessment of children's distress during painful medical procedures. *Health Psychol.*, **2**:133–47.
26. Katz E. R., Kellerman J., Siegal S. E. (1980). Behavioral distress in children with cancer undergoing medical procedures: Developmental considerations. *J. Consult. Clin. Psychol.*, **48**:356–65.
27. Owen M. E. , Todt E. H. (1984). Pain in infancy: Neonatal reaction to a heel lance. *Pain*, **20**:77–86.
28. McGrath P. J., Johnson G., Goodman J. T., Schillinger J., Dunn J., Chapman J. (1987). The Children's Hospital of Eastern Ontario Pain Scale (CHEOPS): A behavioral scale to measure postoperative pain in children. In: Fields H. L., Dubner R., Cevero F., eds. *Advances in pain, research and therapy. Vol. 9*. New York: Raven Press 395–402.
29. Varni J. W., Walco G. A., Katz E. R. (1989). Assessment and management of chronic and recurrent pain in children with chronic diseases. *Pediatrician*, **16**:56–63.
30. Arunasalam K., Davenport H. T., Painter S., Jones J. G. (1983). Ventilatory response to morphine in young and old subjects. *Anaesthesia*, **38**:529–33.
31. McCafferty M., Wong D. L. (1993). Nursing interventions for pain control in children. In: Schechter N. L., Berde C. B., Yaster M., eds. *Pain in infants, children, and adolescents*. Baltimore: Williams & Wilkins, 295–316.
32. Miller R. R., Jick H. (1978). Clinical effects of meperidine in hospitalized medical patients. *J. Clin. Pharmacol.*, **18**:180–9.
33. Beasley S. W., Tibballs J. (1987). Efficacy and safety of continuous morphine infusion for postoperative analgesia in the pediatric surgical ward. *Aust. N. Z. J. Surg.*, **57**:233–7.
34. Dilworth N. M., MacKellar A. (1987). Pain relief for the pediatric surgical patient. *J. Pediatr. Surg.*, **22**:264–6.
35. Shannon M., Berde C. B. (1989). Pharmacologic management of pain in children and adolescents. *Pediatr. Clin. North. Am.*, **36**:855–871.
36. Schechter N. L., Allen D. (1986). Physicians' attitudes toward pain in children. *J. Dev. Behav. Pediatr.*, 350–4.
37. Chapman C. R., Hill H. R. (1989). Prolonged morphine self-administration and addiction liability. *Cancer*, 1636–44.
38. Morrison R. A. (1991). Update on sickle cell disease: incidence of addition and choice of opioid in pain management. *Pediatr. Nurs.*, **17**:503.
39. Pegelow C. H. (1992). Survey of pain management therapy provided for children with sickle cell disease. *Clin. Pediatr.*, **31**:211–4.
40. Angell M. (1982). The quality of mercy. *N. Engl. J. Med.*, **306**:98–9.
41. Berde C., Ablin A., Glazer J, *et al.*, (1990). Report of the Subcommittee on Disease-Related Pain in Childhood Cancer. *Pediatrics*, **86**:S818–S825.
42. Zeltzer L. K., Altman A., Cohen D., *et al.*, (1990). Report of the Subcommittee on the Management of Pain Associated with Procedures in Children with Cancer. *Pediatrics*, **86**:S826–S831.
43. American Pain Society (1992). *Principles of analgesic use in the treatment of acute pain and cancer pain*, 3rd ed.Skokie, IL.
44. Agency for Health Care Policy and Research (1992). Acutepain management: Operative or medical procedures and trauma. Rockville, MD: US Department of Health and Human Services.

12 Ethical Issues in Pediatric Organ Transplantation

Joel E. Frader

Children's Hospital of Pittsburgh, 3705 Fifth Avenue at De Soto Street, Pittsburg, PA 15213, USA

INTRODUCTION

By the early 1990s, organ transplantation reached into every field of medical and surgical practice. With the phenomenal growth of transplantation, physicians, patients, family members, hospital administrators, and society in general have had to come to grips quickly with a host of associated ethical problems. This chapter discusses the range of moral challenges raised by transplant therapies used for children.

MEDICAL OVERVIEW

Bone

Allograft bone transplants are used to treat bone tumors, major skeletal defects and in other kinds of plastic/reconstructive surgery. The processing of bone for transplants provides a mechanical matrix with relatively little antigenicity.[1] Bone transplantation, in and of itself, raises few ethical concerns.

Bone marrow

Bone marrow transplantation (BMT) has become relatively frequent in the treatment of various childhood cancers. The technique has also emerged as a principal therapy for primary immunodeficiencies, aplastic anemia, some storage diseases, and hemoglobinopathies. There has been some controversy over children serving as bone marrow donors,[2,3,4] but the major moral problem involves the appropriateness of BMT for diseases which have long and variable courses. The problem lies in the substantial risks,[5] including death from primary graft failure, overwhelming infection prior to reconstitution of immune function, acute and chronic graft-versus-host disease, and cancer.

Cardiac

Surgeons now perform cardiac transplantation in children for congenital heart diseases, like hypoplastic left heart syndrome (HLHS), not readily ameliorated by corrective procedures. The other major indication is end-stage cardiomyopathy. As with most other solid organ transplants, the ethical problems include the long-term burdens of immunosuppression, especially recurrent infection and malignancy, and rejection. The latter apparently poses a particular problem with cardiac grafts, namely the risk of arrhythmia and sudden death.[6,7] Rapidly progressive, drug-induced coronary artery disease has also been a hardship.[8]

Cardiac–lung

Combined cardiac–lung transplantation attempts to treat those with primary lung disease or pulmonary vascular hypertension with irreversible cardiac failure. The most common disorder leading to heart–lung transplantation in children is cystic fibrosis. The most prominent ethical problem surrounding heart–lung transplantation stems from the reported intermediate-term survival (27–52% at two years).[9,10,11]

Cardiac valves and major vessels

Thoracic surgeons also use cardiac valves and other vascular structures procured from cadavers and processed to prevent infection and prolong shelf-life. These allografts usually provide superior function and fit compared to either mechanical devices or xenografts. There has been recent speculation that premature and/or abrupt allograft failure actually represents acute rejection (personal communication, Ralph Siewers, M.D.). Proof of such claims should lead to improved informed consent about the risks (and benefits) of vascular allografts.

Corneas

Corneal transplantation is well established for problems of corneal opacity. Technical considerations may limit the treatment in the very young. Treatment rarely involves major systemic immunosuppression.

Gastrointestinal

Among the newest transplantation efforts are those involving the gastrointestinal tract, particularly the use of the small bowel, with or without associated liver or pancreas transplantation. Early attempts at bowel transplantation met with serious difficulties with translocation of bacteria, resulting in sepsis, and with graft-versus-host disease from bowel-associated lymphoid tissue. The initial results were so discouraging that they led one renowned transplant surgeon to call for a moratorium on the practice until laboratory investigation offered more promise of success.[12] As of mid-1993, revised surgical techniques, graft preparation, recipient antibiotic treatment, and altered immunosuppressive regimens have improved results, though these transplants remain experimental in the eyes of most.[13,14]

Success in small bowel transplantation holds particular promise for children with short-gut syndrome from congenital abnormalities or extensive resections for necrotizing enterocolitis. Many of these children, treated with total parenteral nutrition, have associated liver injury, and may benefit from combined intestinal–liver transplantation. We have no meaningful information about the intermediate- or long-term outcomes regarding survival, graft function, ability of the patients to eat adequately, major complications, or quality of life. In addition, the treatment is extremely expensive.

Kidney

Kidney transplantation represents the treatment of choice for end-stage renal disease in children.[15] In all but the smallest children, graft and recipient survival approach those in adults. Controversy continues regarding the need for matching by tissue type which, in turn, affects access to kidneys for those without available living donors.[16,17] The distribution of tissue types in the population follows ethnic and racial lines. Thus, insistence on tissue type-matched organs reduces the potential pool of kidneys for members of minority communities.[18,19]

Liver

Liver transplantation became the second "routine" organ replacement therapy in children in the early 1980s with the introduction of cyclosporine–steroid immunosuppression. Since then, the most common indication for childhood liver transplantation has been biliary atresia. Some acute conditions also trigger consideration of transplantation, including fulminant hepatic failure from toxic causes, non-Hepatitis B viral infections, and Wilson's disease. Chronic problems associated with cirrhosis and a few genetic disorders include liver failure and/or life-threatening portal hypertension with gastrointestinal bleeding. One-and five year survival now exceed 80% in some centers and for many children the quality of life improves substantially after successful transplantation.[20–22] Indications for liver transplantation remain somewhat controversial. For instance, Starzl and colleagues have suggested liver transplantation for some inborn metabolic disorders.[23] In at least one, glucose-6-phosphatase deficiency (Type I glycogen storage disease), however, there may be no intrinsic liver disease and the metabolic derangements of early life can be treated with night-time continuous enteral feeding, avoiding the invasiveness and long-term risks of transplantation.

Lung

Lung transplantation has taken somewhat longer to become established than combined heart–lung operations. Technical advances and the desire to make hearts available separately have recently spurred enthusiasm for transplantation of the lungs alone.[24] In children, the single most frequent indication is cystic fibrosis. Acute and chronic rejection appears to be a major problem for transplantation involving the lungs and currently limits the prognosis. Persistent life-threatening infection with unusual and/or resistant micro-organisms has plagued patients transplanted for cystic fibrosis.

Pancreas

Pancreas transplantation has not enjoyed widespread use in the treatment of children. Whole pancreas or islet cell transplantation remains experimental.[25,26]

ORGAN AVAILABILITY AND PROCUREMENT

While not a moral problem in and of itself, the lack of organs able to be used for clinical transplantation in children results in substantial numbers of deaths among those awaiting organ replacement. As a consequence, voluntary organizations, like groups of parents whose children need or have had transplants, procurement agencies, and physicians caring for the children have focused a great deal of attention on increasing the supply of transplantable organs. Efforts in this regard have included educational programs for the public and health care personnel to increase awareness of the need for and value of organs from children who have injuries or illness resulting in brain death. (Unfortunately, it sometimes seems interested parties pay more attention to organ procurement issues than to primary prevention of accidents and injuries through such measures as seat belt or bicycle helmet use.)

Despite earlier fears, available evidence now suggests that the criteria for diagnosing brain death in children, except perhaps in the first week of life, do not differ substantively from those used with adults.[27] Clinical experience[28] and opinion surveys[29] in the United States and Canada suggest that most parents believe they would donate organs if faced with the brain death of their child. Actual donation rates from parents of brain dead minor children may be somewhat higher than the rates from relatives of adults suffering the same fate. No evidence suggests parents harbor anger or resentment against pediatricians, neurosurgeons, or others who request organ donation, despite the fears of many health care providers.

The push to procure more organs to supply the ever-growing demand has led to worry that physicians treating critically ill or injured patients might (even though unaware) alter their care to maximize the likelihood of organ donation, rather than serve the best interests of the patient.[30] This kind of concern led to provisions of the Uniform Anatomical Gift Act that forbid transplant team members from participation in decisions about potential donors. While such apprehension continues, no data provide evidence of widespread compromise of patients' interests.

The shortage of organs has prompted considerable effort to increase potential sources of organs. State and federal laws now require hospitals to ensure that doctors, nurses, or organ procurement personnel approach appropriate surrogates of dead or dying patients and discuss the possibility of organ and/or tissue donation. (Physicians may decide to waive the request for donation if specific medical conditions provide a contra-indication to organ use, such as uncontrolled bacteremia or metastatic cancer.) The implementation of "required request" laws was initially associated with a drop in the rates of organ donation, contrary to their purpose. Improved training in the art of such peri-mortem conversations and a shift in responsibility for conducting the discussions from physicians to specially trained, designated professionals have been associated with increased procurement, though organ shortages persist. Some have suggested further legal changes to allow either "presumed consent" or incentives for family members to donate.[31,32,33,34]

Presumed consent, as permitted by law in some countries, allows removal of organs for transplantation unless patients previously indicated they would not wish to become donors or unless family members object. The rates of organ harvest where such laws now exist have not been dramatically higher than in the United States, apparently because physicians still inquire of and defer to family members. Some feel that presumed consent, given the great diversity in religious attitudes toward and personal beliefs about dead bodies found in the United States, would risk widespread offense.[35]

Incentives to improve donation might include direct cash payments to donor families, coverage of the deceased's funeral costs, or schemes to provide future priority treatment of family members, should they be in need of organs for transplantation. Besides adding to the cost of transplantation,[36] opposition to such proposals involves concern about both the undermining of our system of voluntary, charitable giving and the possibility of coercion or exploitation of patients' families.[37]

Finally, a debate about using anencephalic infants as a source of organs has gone on for decades.[38,39,40] Enthusiasm for obtaining organs from anencephalic babies has somewhat waned recently with declining numbers of live-born infants with this diagnosis, with published re-assessment of the likely number of usable organs (i.e., those unaffected by other congenital defects),[41] and with the unsuccessful "experiment" at Loma Linda University to provide life support until brain death occurred, at which time organs could be procured. That effort resulted in unacceptable prolongation of the dying of the babies and was abandoned.[42]

NON-HEART-BEATING DONATION

Two new attempts, so far limited to adults, to obtain organs have emerged in the early 1990's. The first, in use by the Regional Organ Bank of Illinois, involves patients brought "dead-on-arrival" to or dying in emergency departments.[43] After unsuccessful resuscitations, physicians insert special catheters and begin abdominal and retroperitoneal organ cooling and perfusion with preservation solutions and then seek family permission to procure organs from their deceased relative. As of mid-1993, most families provided consent for the requested donation.

In the second effort, begun at the University of Pittsburgh, organ procurement is tied to elective withdrawal of life support.[44] In the Pittsburgh plan, patients or family members, not health care personnel, must initiate a discussion of organ donation *after* a decision has been made to withdraw life support. If the patient can be a donor, he or she is taken to an operating room where intensive care physicians stop life-sustaining devices and/or drugs. Once the heart has stopped for two minutes, a doctor pronounces death and organ recovery begins. Controversial aspects of this system include: (1) the question of whether two minutes is an adequate "test" of cardiac death;[45] (2) concern about potential conflicts of interest, at least in institutions where transplantation plays a large clinical or research role;[46] and (3) concern about the adverse effects on the family as a result of the patient's death in an operating room, removed from the loved ones.[47]

According to Lynn,[45] while the legal definition of death has included the notion that either brain or cardiac function have ceased *irreversibly*, in practice no one has needed to pay precise attention to the matter. But now, Lynn argues, much hinges on whether the potential non-heart-beating donor is really dead. If the heart can support circulation again, one would have a live patient from whom one could not, legally, and should not, ethically, remove organs. If the heart has stopped irreversibly, one has a cadaver from which procurement may proceed. According to Lynn, we really do not know if a two-minute waiting period signifies cardiovascular death. One could counter, however, that while the distinction may have legal importance, it has no moral weight. After all, in these cases, patients or their surrogates and physicians have already agreed that withdrawal of life support is appropriate and the patient's death is acceptable, even, in some sense, desirable. If this is true, we should consider changing laws which present impediments to this rational, humane goal.

Frader[46] has pointed out that institutions with substantial transplant programs, and their staffs, have dual interests in caring for potential non-heart-beating donors. On the one hand, those caring for such patients have clear obligations to provide life-sustaining and life-enhancing treatment consistent with patients' or surrogates' values. On the other hand, many in the institution benefit from transplantation: patients have a chance at a better life, physicians sustain clinical and training programs through continued transplant activities, and many take advantage of myriad research opportunities associated with transplantation. Thus, personal, academic, and economic rewards come from a thriving transplant program. To the extent that non-heart-beating donors can help sustain transplantation, especially in the face of a growing organ shortage, the institution and its staff have an interest in encouraging non-heart-beating donation.

While the current policy at the University of Pittsburgh Medical Center prohibits staff-initiated discussion of non-heart-beating donation, staff might unconsciously provide non-verbal cues to patients or surrogates to raise the issue. To the degree that institutional and personal identities are tied to transplantation, personnel may, inadvertently, act in ways that foster withdrawal of treatment and organ donation, rather than promote efforts to extend care for those at the margin of survival.

Finally, the current requirements for declaration of death and immediate organ procurement in the operating room may have unintended and negative consequences for family members. This may have special significance in pediatrics. While we have no data on this subject, it is surely the case that many physicians and nurses believe that parents should have the opportunity to be with and hold their dying infants and children. Many parents request the opportunity and in many hospitals personnel regularly offer parents the chance to touch or embrace their son or daughter at the time life-support is discontinued. Separation of the parents from the child's body prior to transfer to the operating room and death may prove psychologically harmful.

However, at least in the Pediatric Intensive Care Unit at the Children's Hospital of Pittsburgh, when physicians and parents agree to withdraw life support, parents frequently ask about the possibility of their child becoming an organ donor. For such families, the act of donation, even if it means the child's death in the operating room, may prove a sufficient, even overriding, compensatory benefit. If non-heart-beating donation from children becomes a reality, pediatricians should seek a systematic study of the impact of parent–child separation at the time of death.

LIVING-RELATED DONATION

Living-related kidney donation permitted the development of renal, and subsequently all modern solid-organ, transplantation. Debate continues in the transplantation community about the superiority, if any, of intermediate- or long-term results with living-related kidneys. For some children, receiving an organ from a relative may offer the only reasonably rapid solution to the rigors of remaining on chronic dialysis. In bone marrow transplantation, sibling donation of tissue type-matched marrow may offer far-and-away the best medical alternative for success. Many centers thus rely on parents or siblings to donate kidneys or marrow to children.

Using minor siblings for kidney and marrow donation raises two important issues. The first concerns the potential medical harms of donation. While there have been few deaths and major perioperative morbidity has been extremely low, a debate continues about whether those with only a single remaining kidney have long-term medical risks, especially of so-called hyperfiltration injury.[48,49] In marrow transplantation the long-term risk to the donor is nil, but must be weighed against the low risks of anesthetic catastrophes and the fears some children may have as a result of blood drawing, intravenous line insertion, hospitalization, post-operative pain, and so on.

The second issue has to do with consent. Earlier in the history of transplantation, physicians turned to the courts for review and protection when considering removal of a solid organ or bone marrow from a child donor.[50,51] Now, it seems, physicians and families, sometimes with the help of ethics consultants or ethics committees, consider the following: (1) the decision-making capacity of a minor who may become a donor; (2) the benefits and burdens of donation; (3) whether parents in a particular case have conflicts of interest which interfere with their making a decision for each involved child; and (4) whether consent can be given voluntarily under the stress of a sibling's life-threatening illness.

Consent for donation by a minor child depends on both the law in a particular jurisdiction and the maturity of the potential child-donor.[52] Children judged mature by a court, and/or children considered emancipated under state law may consent to become organ donors without parental permission, though most would agree on the desirability of family accord on such an important subject. The act of donation may or may not provide psychological benefit to siblings. Curran argues that preventing a child from donating to a brother or sister may produce irreparable harm.[53] It is also possible that subtle coercion of a child to become a donor could produce lasting psychological damage.

Finally, the issue of voluntariness in family donations has not received explicit attention with respect to children. In situations involving adult donors, sociologists[54,55] have documented intense familial pressure for donation and at least one surgeon has expressed grave reservations about relatives' freedom to refuse to donate.[56] It simply is not clear how one would prevent unconscious or explicit pressure on a sibling who might be a donor, nor is it entirely clear it would be ethically or psychologically appropriate to do so. That is to say, families may be justified in urging one sibling to donate to another, and the line between appropriate encouragement and undue coercion is extremely difficult to draw. Here too, we need serious empirical study of the consequences of actual practice.

A particularly interesting set of questions arises with regard to the donation of segments of non-paired organs, namely liver, lung, and pancreas from live donors. The ethical issues involved in the first two have been discussed recently.[57,58] In the limited experience so far, only adults have served as donors. The perioperative morbidity has been low. There have been no reported deaths. Available evidence suggests that the body will regenerate most, if not all, resected liver mass. Lung tissue does not regenerate. The latter may have important implications for the recipient as well as the donor. That is, adult lung segments may not adapt to being in a child's body and the recipients may outgrow the volume of transplanted lung, leading to respiratory insufficiency and the need for another transplant.

In any case, the major ethical problem here seems to be that of expectations placed upon potential donors. If these procedures have reasonable technical success and the shortage of cadaver donors remains, we need to worry about the internal and external pressures placed upon prospective donors who may have a host of responsibilities and feelings which would make major surgery and its risks difficult to undertake. Perhaps, as with the informal system that has arisen in renal transplantation, we will have to develop a mechanism to conceal a person's eligibility to donate from family members in order to preserve an individual's freedom to decline actual donation. We should not assume that parents (or siblings) have a duty to undergo surgical risks, even to save the life of a child.

XENOGRAFTS

The use of nonhuman live organs has received a great deal of attention since 1984 with the Baby Fae case at Loma Linda University and the subsequent attempted baboon liver transplants at the University of Pittsburgh. As of mid-1993, xenografts have not worked in the clinical situations where surgeons have tried them. Many in the transplant community seem confident that progress in immunosuppressive therapy will ultimately permit successful xenografting.[59,60]

Even if science conquers the immunologic barriers, several important issues remain. First, do nonhuman animals, perhaps especially primates, have rights or interests which would limit their sacrifice for human transplantation purposes? For those inclined to answer affirmatively, one should consider the implications of this for current research programs, such as those that infect chimpanzees with HIV, where primates are harmed or killed in the name of saving human lives. Second, the possibility exists that infecting or colonizing organisms in the primate donor, especially viruses, could infect immunosuppressed human organ recipients (even if the same microbes would be harmless to a normal host).[61] While medical science can now identify and test for some of these microorganisms, we may find new ones, previously unknown to us, only after they harm transplant recipients.

ORGAN ALLOCATION

Current allocation schemes vary depending on the organ or organs involved. Time on the waiting list, urgency of need (usually tied to receipt of intensive care), blood and tissue matching, and so on, all contribute to determining who gets an available organ. In 1991 the semi-public United Network for Organ Sharing (UNOS), which regulates organ procurement and distribution in the United States, mandated a so-called "local use" policy which requires organs be used, if at all possible, within the geographic area covered by the organ procurement agency recovering the organ. The policy is supposed to encourage further donation by helping the community see the fruits of transplantation, reduce organ waste brought about by the ischemia associated with long-distance organ transportation, and save money spent on transporting organs to distant centers. In addition, the policy rests on the claim that organ use by small local or regional hospitals is as successful as in the major transplant centers.

The major centers opposed the change from the previous distribution policy, which had tended to allocate more organs to the large-volume programs. The new policy made fewer organs available to big centers, decreasing the number of operations they could perform, increasing the deaths of their patients awaiting transplants, and "penalized" the centers which accepted higher risk patients for treatment.

A serious social concern has been raised by many who have noted that minority members have relatively limited access to transplant services.[62,63,64] The reasons for this are complex and include: (1) limited access to medical care generally, which affects diagnosis and referral in time for transplantation to be a realistic option; (2) relative infrequency of tissue types within minority communities, limiting access to tissue-type-matched organs; (3) prejudice (conscious or otherwise) in organ distribution; and (4) cultural factors that may make minority members reluctant to undergo available transplantation.

Other concerns have also arisen about competition between those awaiting single organs and those waiting to receive multiple organs (hearts or lungs vs heart–lungs, livers or bowel vs liver–bowel, etc). "Efficiency" considerations might suggest that distributing single organs would allow the largest number of waiting patients to benefit. But, rules maximizing the number of recipients would, given the overall shortage of organs, effectively eliminate multi-organ transplantation, denying treatment to an entire class of patients. On the other hand, rules giving multi-organ recipients priority removes relatively large numbers of organs from the distribution pool.

All of this sharply highlights the fact that we have no clarity about the most appropriate moral grounds for deciding how to distribute organs. Some policies favor transplanting the sickest patients, who tend to have poorer prognoses even with transplantation. Such an approach satisfies our desire to try to rescue those in the most dire straits. But, this conflicts with other notions of fairness that favor "productivity", here meaning the maximizing of organ (and patient) survival, which would call for selecting the healthier candidates. Other policies would attempt to correct for present or past discrimination, whether based on racial, economic, or other factors. The point here is that there are principled ethical differences about how to allocate scarce resoures like organs for transplantation, and no clear consensus on how to order the "perfect" organ distribution plan.

EXPERIMENTATION, INNOVATION, AND STANDARDS OF CARE

While most agree that physicians must adhere to higher standards for consent and conduct in experimental situations than under "accepted" therapeutic circumstances, there is less clarity about what actually constitutes clinical experimentation or innovation. Levine attempted to distinguish between these on the basis of intent, saying that experimentation entails production of generalizable knowledge, while novel efforts primarily to help patients involve *nonvalidated practice*.[65] No matter what the appropriate phrase, it is sometimes difficult to discern whether or when a particular set of transplantation activities has moved from experimentation or innovation to "routine" practice. The distinction has more than philosophical importance. Different designations create significant differences in the standards for information disclosure in the consent process, in whether procedures are reimburseable, and in the discretion we allow parents to accept or refuse proposed treatments.[66]

The medical and technical issues in transplantation are changing rapidly and therefore provide a target moving too rapidly to pin down here. Can we say easily that organ replacement for any given condition is so well established that it represents a standard of care which, like penicillin for meningococcal meningitis, parents may not ordinarily refuse? Could the parents of a young child and their primary care pediatrician legitimately agree to forgo subspecialty evaluation regarding transplant suitability in cases where organ replacement offers the only treatment besides palliation?[67]

As a general rule, we might want to say that the more beneficial the treatment and the fewer the alternatives, the more parents would have an obligation to accept it. But, this only begs the question; we still have to decide what constitutes *sufficient* benefit (and sufficiently small burdens) to trigger a judgment that treatment is morally required. We might want to say that, under most circumstances, *renal* transplantation (and no other type) falls into the ethically obligatory category, compared to either chronic dialysis or death. Usually, the personal, social, and medical quality of life with a kidney transplant exceeds that experienced with continuous ambulatory dialysis or machine-based dialysis several days a week. We would certainly have questions about the judgment of parents who preferred dialysis for their child. Such a preference would almost certainly lead to a serious examination of the decision-making abilities of the parents.

But, what of parents who refuse liver transplantation for a child with progressive cirrhosis several years after a Kasai operation for biliary atresia? Assume the parents have had contact with other patients with similar problems (and their parents) at the time of follow-up visits to the pediatric gastro-enterologist and surgeons. Assume also that the parents have acquired a reasonable familiarity with the literature on transplantation and with the experience of families that have elected that option. With all of this, the parents conclude they do not want to subject their 4-year-old to the risks of transplant surgery and its various post-operative complications. They feel, based on what they have seen and heard from families and physicians and what they have read, that the chance of an 85% one-year actuarial survival for their child does not tell an adequate story. Too many of the transplanted children they have seen have suffered too much, in their view, and they have concluded their son would be better off with a peaceful death (assuming the cooperation of their pediatrician in providing appropriate sedation and analgesia).

Different physicians, ethicists, lawyers, child advocates, etc., would likely have different responses to this situation.[68] While the medical community and United States society at large seem to feel liver transplantation provides "routine" treatment for end-stage biliary atresia (and is therefore neither experimental nor innovative), not everyone would say that the burdens of liver transplantation are so minimal that parents such as those described should be taken to court to have their decision-making authority challenged. Liver transplantation may not provide such a clear good that parents should be denied their right to control treatment choices for their child. Similarly, most pediatricians and pediatric cardiologists would not seek court-ordered treatment for parents refusing transplantation for HLHS.

But, the story can become more complex. What if the parents of either the patient with complications of biliary atresia or the child with HLHS indicated their decision rested not solely on a view that transplantation imposed excessive burdens on the child, but that the economic and psychosocial costs of transplantation would pose too heavy a hardship on the rest of the family? Nothing else about the stories differs except the *reasons* the parents offer. Moreover, everyone involved agrees that the stated reasons have substantial validity and reflect genuine concern about the patient as well as the rest of the family. Should we oppose the "right" conclusion if it is reached for the "wrong" reasons?

This discussion cannot provide definitive answers for these complex questions. Suffice it to say that the status of a particular form of transplantation — experimental, innovative, or accepted practice — is often unclear. Even when some, (especially those involved in the practice), believe they have established a clinical standard and consequent ethical obligation, others, (especially primary care physicians and the lay public), may not attach the same moral weight to the standard of care. At this point, perhaps our best strategy is to maintain open minds and substantial flexibility in our approach to these dilemmas.

TRANSPLANTATION RESOURCES

The costs of transplantation can be viewed from several perspectives. While many procedures have high absolute dollar figures associated with them, when those charges are amortized over life-years gained (or better, over improved-quality life-years gained) or over the entire population, some view the cost/benefit ratio as clearly worthwhile.[69] Such calculations, of course, favor transplantation in children, compared to adults. Others feel that the money spent on transplantation would have an even greater beneficial effect if applied instead to preventive programs. Resolution of these disputes awaits better data about the long-term well-being of transplant patients and some societal agreement about what constitutes a fair balance of resource allocation between prevention and health maintenance and chronic medical care, and rescue interventions like transplantation. In the meantime, we should consider one other implication of our increasing use of transplantation technology.

Because transplantation is often very expensive and because many in the United States have no or minimal health insurance, families frequently face a situation where a medically appropriate candidate for some form of transplantation is economically barred from the treatment. (This is true even with some well-insured families with respect to the newer and less established procedures.) While families, transplant centers, and surgeons have begun to aggressively fight denial of coverage by insurance companies and government agencies, these efforts do not always succeed and may take months or years. Unable to come up with the monetary deposits required by hospitals, desperate families may find themselves turned into fund-raising agencies, organizing charity events, promoting media appeals for donations, and developing job-, church-, school-, and social club-based money drives. These activities can become an obsession, diverting time and energy away from the sick child, (as well as other family members), just as the patient's condition deteriorates and parental support may be needed most. While such a distortion of parental roles for the sake of money for medical care has no necessary tie to transplantation (i.e., the same could happen for expensive plastic surgery for congenital craniofacial anomalies, for example), the increasing frequency of transplantation and its "cutting edge" nature bring the economic pressures produced by modern medicine into bold and disturbing relief.

SUMMARY

Organ transplantation raises all of the usual ethical concerns about pediatric practice, including those having to do with the difficulties of surrogate decision-making, the development of the child's ability to agree (assent or consent) to treatment, resource allocation, and so on. Transplantation also highlights the ethical difficulties encountered when medical science attempts to move to a new level of sophistication, converting a biological tragedy into a biotechnical triumph. When medical innovation and research move at the rapid pace that has characterized transplantation, the distinctions between research activities and therapeutic practice can become rather muddled, with physicians, parents, and children all somewhat confused about the precise goals of pressing on in the face of desperate odds. Such practices as non-heart-beating organ procurement, xenotransplantation, and intestinal or lung transplantation which have unproven or marginal clinical efficacy should make us pause and question the price we ask children and their families to pay for the sake of medical progress.

There has been one reported death of a living-related liver segment donor.[70] Also, the issue of permission for medical intervention with children has recently received extensive and important reconsideration.[71]

References

1. Friedlaender, G. E. (1989). Bone grafting and transplantation. In *Principles of Orthopaedic Practice*, edited by R. Dee, E. Mango, and L.C. Hurst, pp. 74–79. New York: McGraw Hill.

2. Serota, F. T., August, C. S., O'Shea, A. T., Woodward, W. T., and Koch, P. A. (1981). Role of a child advocate in the selection of donors for pediatric bone marrow transplantation. *J. Pediatr.*, **98**:847–850.
3. Williams, T. E. (1984). Legal issues and ethical dilemmas surrounding bone marrow transplantation in children. *Am. J. Pediatr. Hematol/Oncol.*, **6**:83–88.
4. Curran, W. J. (1991). Beyond the best interests of a child: bone marrow transplantaion among half-siblings. *N. Engl. J.Med.*, **324**:1818–1819.
5. Dopfer, R. and Niethammner, D. (1993). Report on the international workshop of the Kind Philipp Foundation on late effects after bone marrow transplantation in childhood malignancies. *Pediatr. Hematol. Oncol.*, 10:63–84.
6. Pahl, E., Fricker, F. J., Trento, A., Griffith, B., Hardesty, R., Gold, L., *et al.*, (1988). Late follow-up of children after heart transplantation. *Transplant. Proc.* **20**(suppl 1):743–746.
7. Heublein, B., Haverich, A., and Borst, H. G. (1990). Long-term follow-up after orthotopic heart transplantation. *Thorac. Cariovasc. Surg.* **38**:285–290.
8. Pahl, E., Fricker, F. J., Armitage, J., Griffith, B. P., Taylor, S., Uretsky, B. F., *et al.*, (1990). Coronary arteriosclerosis in pediatric heart transplant survivors: limitation of long-term survival. *J. Pediatr.*, **116**:177–183.
9. Warner, J. O. (1991). Heart–lung transplantation: all the facts. *Arch. Dis. Child.*, **66**:1013–1017.
10. Starnes, V. A., Marshall, S. E., Lewiston, N. J., Theodore, J., Stinson, E. B., and Shumway, N. E. (1991). Heart–lung transplantation in infants, children, and adolescents. *J. Pediatr. Surg.*, **26**:434–438.
11. Madden, B. P., Hodson, M. E., Tsang, V., Radley-Smith, R., Haghani, A., and Yacoub, M. Y. (1992). Intermediate-term results of heart–lung transplantation for cystic fibrosis. *Lancet*, **339**:1583–1587.
12. Moore, F. D. (1989). The desperate case: CARE (Costs, Applicability, Research, Ethics). *JAMA*, **261**:1483–1484.
13. Todo, S., Tzakis, A. G., Abu-Elmagd, K., Reyes, J., Fung, J., Casavilla, A, *et al.*, (1992). Cadaveric small bowel and small bowel–liver transplantation in humans. *Transplantation*, **53**:369–376.
14. Clark, C. I. (1992). Recent progress in intestinal transplantation. *Arch. Dis. Child.*, **67**:976–979.
15. Morel, P., Almond, P. S., Matas, A. J., Gillingham, K. J., Chau, C., Brown, A., *et al.*, (1991). Long-term quality of life after kidney transplantation in children. *Transplantation*, **52**:47–53.
16. Burdick, J. F., Diethelm, A., Thompson, J. S., Van Buren, C. T., and Williams, G. M. (1991). Organ sharing — present realities and future possibilities. *Transplantation*, **51**:287–292.
17. Burkus, D. E., Meydrech, E. F., and Raju, S. S. (1992). Racial differences in the survival of cadaveric renal allografts: overriding effects of HLA matching and socioeconomic factors. *N. Engl. J. Med.*, **327**:840–845.
18. Kjellstrand, C. M. (1988). Age, sex, and race inequality in renal transplantation. *Arch. Intern. Med.*, **148**:1305–1309.
19. Kasiske, B. L., Neylan, J. F., Riggio, R. R., Danovitch, G. M., Kahana, L., Alexander, S. R., *et al.*, (1991). The effect of race on access and outcome in transplantation. *N. Engl. J. Med.*, **324**:302–307.
20. Zitelli, B. J., Miller, J. W., Gartner, J. C., Malatack, J. J., Urbach, A. H., Belle, S. H., *et al.*, (1988). Changes in life-style after liver transplantation. *Pediatrics*, **82**:173–180.
21. Whitington, P. F. and Balistreri, W. F. (1991). Liver transplantation in pediatrics: indications, contraindications, and pretransplant management. *J. Pediatr.*, **118**:169–177.
22. Salt, A., Noble-Jamieson, G., Barnes, N. D., Mowat, A. P., Rolles, K., Jamieson, N., *et al.*, (1992). Liver transplantation in 100 children: Cambridge and King's College Hospital series. *Brit. Med. J.*, **304**:416–21.
23. Starzl, T. E., Demetris, A. J., and Van Thiel, D. (1989). Liver transplantation. *N. Engl. J. Med.*, **321**:1014–1022.
24. Bonser, R. S., Fragomeni, L. S., Kriett, J. M., Kaye, M. P., and Jamieson, S. W. (1988). Technique of clinical double-lung transplantation. *J. Heart Transplant.*, **7**:293–303.
25. Allen, D. B. and MacDonald, M. J. (1990). Pancras and islet cell transplantation for type I diabetes mellitus: does it have a role for children? *Adv. Pediatr.*, **37**:391–412.

26. Drash, A. L. and Arslanian, S. A. (1990). Can insulin-dependent diabetes mellitus be cured or prevented? A status report on immunomodulatory strategies and pancreas transplantation. *Pediatr. Clin. N. Amer.,* **37**:1467–87.
27. Special Task Force. (1987). Guidelines for the determination of brain death in children. *Pediatrics,* **80**:298–300.
28. Morris, J. A., Wilcox, T. R., and Frist, W. H. (1992). Pediatric organ donation: the paradox of organ shortage despite the remarkable willingness of families to donate. *Pediatrics,* **89**:411–415.
29. Walker, J. A., McGraft, P. J., MacDonald, N. E., Wells, G., Petrusic, W., and Nolan, B. E. (1990). Parental attitudes toward pediatric organ donation: a survey. *Can. Med. Assoc. J.,* **142**:1383–1387.
30. Caplan, A. L. (1992). Requests, gifts, and obligations: the ethics of organ procurement. In: Caplan, A. L. *If I Were A Rich Man Could I Buy a Pancreas*? Bloomington, Indiana: Indiana University Press.
31. Sanders, L. M., Devney, P., Young, E., Raffin, T. A. (1992). The organ donation committee: an ethically responsible approach to increasing the organ donation rate. *Chest,* **102**:1572–77.
32. Peters, T. G. (1991) Life or death: the issue of payment in cadaveric organ donation. *JAMA,* **265**:1302–1305.
33. Pellegrino, E. D. (1991). Families' self-interest and the cadaver's organs: what price consent? *JAMA,* **265**:1305–1306.
34. Kittur, D. S., Hogan M. M., Thukral, V. K., McGaw, L. J., Alexander, J. W. (1991). Incentives for organ donation? *Lancet,* **338**:1441–1443.
35. Youngner, S. J. (1990). Organ retrieval: can we ignore the dark side? *Transplant. Proc.,* **22**:1014–1015.
36. Evans, R. W. (1993). Organ procurement expenditures and the role of financial incentives. *JAMA,* **269**:3113–3118.
37. Peters, D. A. (1986). Protecting autonomy in organ procurement procedures: some overlooked issues. *Milbank Quart.,* **64**:241–270.
38. Martin, L. W., Gonzales, L. L., West, C. D., Swartz, P. A., and Sutorius, D. J. (1969). Homotransplantation of both kidneys from an anencephalic monster to a 17 pound bou with Eagle-Barrett syndrome. *Surgery,* **66**:603–607.
39. Shewmon, D. A., Capron, A. M., Peacock, W. J., and Schulman, B. L., (1989). The use of anencephalic infants as organ sources: a critique. *JAMA,* **261**:1773–1781.
40. Committee on Bioethics of the American Academy of Pediatrics (1992). Infants with anencephaly as organ sources: ethical considerations. *Pediatrics,* **89**:1116–1119.
41. Medical Task Force on Anencephaly (1990). The infant with anencephaly. *N. Engl. J. Med.,* **322**:669–674.
42. Peabody, J. L., Emery, J. R., and Ashwal, S. (1989). Experience with anencephalic infants as prospective organ donors. *N. Engl. J. Med.,* **321**:344–50.
43. De Vita, M. A., Snyder, J. V., and Grenvik, A. (1993). History of organ donation by patients with cardiac death. *Kennedy Institute of Ethics Journal,* **3**:113–129.
44. De Vita, M. A. and Snyder, J. V. (1993). Development of the University of Pittsburgh Medical Center policy for the care of terminally ill patients who may become organ donors after death following the removal of life support. *Kennedy Institute of Ethics Journal,* **3**:131–143.
45. Lynn, J. (1993). Are the patients who become organ donors under the Pittsburgh protocol for "non-heart-beating donors" really dead? *Kennedy Institute of Ethics Journal,* **3**:167–178.
46. Frader, J. (1993). Non-heart-beating organ donation: personal and institutional conflicts of interest. *Kennedy Institute of Ethics Journal,* **3**:189–198.
47. Fox, R. C. (1993). "An ignoble form of cannibalism": reflections on the Pittsburgh protocol for procuring organs from non-heart-beating cadavers. *Kennedy Institute of Ethics Journal,* **3**:231–239.
48. Steckler, R. E., Riehle, R. A., and Vaughan, E. D. (1990). Hyperfiltration-induced renal injury in normal man: myth or reality? *J. Urology,* **144**:1323–1327.

49. Watnick, T. J., Jenkins, R. R., Rackoff, P. Baumgarten, A., and Bia, M. J. (1988). Microalbuminuria and hypertension in long-term renal donors. *Transplantation*, **45**:59–65.
50. Fost, N. (1977). Children as renal donors. *N. Engl. J. Med.*, **296**:363–367.
51. Holder, A.R. (1985). *Legal Issues in Pediatrics and Adolescent Medicine*, 2nd ed. New Haven, Conn: Yale University Press, pp. 146–178.
52. Morrissey, J. M., Hoffman, A. D., and Thrope, J. C. (1986). *Consent and Confidentiality in the Health Care of Children and Adolescents: A Legal Guide*. New York: The Free Press.
53. Curran, W. J. (1991). Beyond the best interests of a child: bone marrow transplantation among half-siblings. *N. Engl. J. Med.*, **324**:1818–1819.
54. Fox, R. C. and Swazey, J. P. (1974). *The Courage to Fail: A Social View of Organ Transplants and Dialysis*. Chicago: University of Chicago Press.
55. Simmons, R. G., Klein, S. D., and Simmons, R. I. (1977). *Gift of Life: The Effects of Organ Transplantation on Individual, Family, and Societal Dynamics*. New York: John Wiley and Sons.
56. Starzl, T. E. (1987). Living donors: con. *Transplant. Proc.*, **19**:174–175.
57. Singer, P. A., Siegler, M., Whitington, P. F., Lantos, J. D., Emond, J. C., Thistlewaite, J. R., *et al.* (1989). Ethics of liver transplantation with living donors. *N. Engl. J. Med.*, **321**:620–622.
58. Shaw, L. R., Miller, J. D., Slutsky, A. S., Maurer, J. R., Puskas, J. D., Patterson, G. A., *et al.*, (1991). Ethics of lung transplantation with live donors. *Lancet*, **338**:678–680.
59. Sells, R. (1992). Bookshelf (Xenotransplantation — The Transplantation of Organs and Tissues Between Species). *Lancet*, **339**:917–918.
60. Starzl, T. E., Fung, J., Tzakis, A., Todo, S., Demetris, A. J., Marino, I. R., *et al.*, (1993). Baboon-to-human liver transplantation. *Lancet*, **341**:65–71.
61. Nowak, R. (1992). Hope or horror? Primate-to-human organ transplants. *J. NIH Research*, **4**(Sept):37–38.
62. Kjellstrand, C. M. (1988). Age, sex, and race inequality in renal transplantation. *Arch. Intern. Med.*, **148**:1305–1309.
63. Held, P. J., Pauly, M. V., Bovbjerg, R. R., Newmann, J., Salvatierra, O. (1988). *Arch. Intern. Med.*, **148**:2594–2600.
64. Kasiske, B. L., Neylan, J. F., Riggio, R. R., Danovitch, G. M., Kahana, L., Alexander, S. R., White, M. G. (1991). The effect of race on access and outcome in transplantation. *N. Engl. J. Med.*, **324**:302–307.
65. Levine, R. J. (1981). *Ethics and Regulation of Clinical Research.* Baltimore, Maryland: Urban & Schwarzenberg.
66. Lantos, J.D. and Frader, J. (1990). Extracorporeal membrane oxygenation and the ethics of clinical research in pediatrics. *N. Engl. J. Med.*, **323**:409–413.
67. Frader, J. (1994). Perilous life-sustaining therapy and the primary care physician: should the buck stop there? *Clin. Pediatr.*, **33**:185–188.
68. Moskop, J. C. (1987). Organ transplantation in children: ethical issues. *J. Pediatr.*, **110**:175–180.
69. Hauboldt, R. H. (1993). Cost implications of human organ transplantations, an update: 1993. *Medical Benefits*, **10**(6) p. 1.
70. Sterneck, M., Nischwitz, U., Fischer, L., Malago, M., Roglers, X., Raedler, A., *et al.*, (1995). Evaluation and morbidity of the living liver donor in pediatric liver transplantation. *Transplant. Proc.*, **27**:1164–1165.
71. Committee on Bioethics, American Academy of Pediatrics. (1995). Informed consent, parental permission, and assent in pediatric practice. *Pediatrics*, **95**:314–317.

13 Trials and Tribulations: The Ethics of Responsible Research

Ruth Macklin

Albert Einstein College of Medicine, 1300 Morris Park Avenue (Belfer Building) Bronx, New York 10461, USA

The objective of all well-designed research is to contribute to scientific understanding. The category of biomedical research known as clinical investigation seeks to gain knowledge about the mechanisms of disease and the efficacy of therapies that might cure, mitigate, or palliate specific diseases. Since these are noble aims, what sorts of ethical problems are posed by the research endeavor? And why do these problems require special attention in the case of children?

Unlike medical therapy, in which physicians employ established treatments designed to benefit their patients, research maneuvers have as yet unproven benefits and possibly unknown risks of harm. The idea of experimenting on patients conjures up two quite different pictures. The first depicts individuals who are sick and suffering — perhaps even dying — being subjected to the manipulations of clinical investigators who use patients in their efforts to contribute to scientific knowledge, as well as to promote their own careers. The second picture portrays untold numbers of present and future patients receiving the benefits of miraculous cures resulting from painstaking research in hospitals and laboratories. Neither of these pictures is an accurate rendering of the actual conduct of research involving human subjects, yet both contain partial truths.

The ethical dilemma created by the need to experiment on sick patients in order to advance the frontiers of biomedical science and conquer disease is sometimes stated in the form of two unacceptable extremes. To allow unfettered experiments on human beings would open up the prospect of new abuses such as those known to have occurred in the past. The atrocities committed by the Nazis in the name of medical research — such as the gruesome experiments performed by Dr. Josef Mengele on children who were identical twins[2] — are the worst example but not the only instance of unethical research conducted on human subjects. However, to prohibit research on human subjects altogether would be to close off the only avenues that could provide the scientific knowledge and technological capabilities for preventing and curing diseases.

The most fundamental ethical requirement for conducting research on human subjects is the need to obtain each subject's voluntary, informed consent to participate. The fundamental status of this requirement derives from the very nature of the moral life, which relies on principles of how people ought to treat one another. Ethical treatment of human beings requires that they not be treated as mere things, like inanimate objects, as instruments to further the ends or purposes of others. The requirement of informed consent to be a subject of research recognizes that it is ethically permissible for people to serve the ends of others, but only if they freely consent to the arrangement and adopt the ends or purposes of others as their own.

This principle was first enunciated in clear and unequivocal language in the Nuremberg Code, which emerged from the trial of Nazi physicians in post-World War II Nuremberg, Germany. Article One of the Code states that "The voluntary consent of the human subject is absolutely essential". Prior to this time there had been no code of ethics governing research involving human subjects. The Nuremberg Code marked the first attempt to formulate ethical principles and detailed provisions enunciating a universal standard to guide the conduct of biomedical research.

To carry out research on people without their knowledge or consent, whether they are normal, healthy individuals or sick patients, violates this fundamental principle. This is where questions about involving children as research subjects begin. Are children capable of granting informed consent? If not, may they be enrolled as research subjects? If they may, according to what ethical principle can their participation be justified? The Nuremberg Code did not mention children as subjects of research, but silence on that point need not be construed as implicit disapproval.

REGULATION OF RESEARCH

Ethical issues regarding children as subjects of biomedical research was first addressed systematically and in depth by the National Commission for the Protection of Human Subjects of Biomedical and Behavioral Research (hereinafter, the National Commission), a commission established in the United States by the National Research Act of 1974.[3] The National Commission was charged with making reports and recommendations in several areas of research involving human subjects. Special attention was paid to vulnerable populations, and one of the Commission's reports was devoted exclusively to research involving children.[4] The Commission's report and recommendations appeared in 1977, but it was not until 1983 that those recommendations were incorporated into the Code of Federal Regulations that applies to federally funded research.[5]

The mechanism that has been adopted to deal with the practical problems of protecting human subjects is regulation of the research enterprise. Procedural safeguards of several kinds are in place to monitor or review the conduct of research on human subjects. Most importantly, every institution that receives funds from the U.S. Department of Health and Human Services (DHHS) for biomedical and behavioral research on human beings is required to have a committee, known as an Institutional Review Board (IRB), to review and approve research protocols before the study is actually begun.[6] Officially required only to review research conducted or funded by DHHS, these committees are now in place virtually everywhere in the United States, including pharmaceutical companies that pay for and carry out their own drug research. Most IRBs — at least those in academic medical centers — are charged with reviewing all research projects conducted in their institutions, whether or not they are funded in whole or in part by grants from DHHS.

Two agencies in the federal government are responsible for overseeing human subjects research. One is the Food and Drug Administration (FDA), whose regulations govern all research on new drugs and devices. The other is an office within the Department of Health and Human Services, the Office for Protection from Research Risks (OPRR), which oversees research conducted in institutions receiving funds from the National Institutes of Health.

Federal regulations governing the conduct of research on human subjects charge Institutional Review Boards with several tasks. The two main functions are first, to ensure that each research protocol has a favorable benefit–risk ratio, and second, to determine that the procedures for obtaining informed consent are adequate. While the risks of human experimentation are always borne by the subjects, the potential benefits are calculated to include others besides the research subjects, such as future patients suffering from the same disease.

The most general protection afforded to children as potential research subjects is the requirement that when possible, the drug, device, or research maneuver must first be tested on adult subjects. Although this requirement serves in many cases to protect children from being initial subjects in an investigation of new drug treatments or in surgical procedures such as organ transplantation, it is clearly inapplicable to much pediatric research. Research directed at extreme prematurity, at diseases unique to children, or seeking to gather baseline data about normal physiologic functioning can only be done on infants and children.

ETHICAL PRINCIPLES FOR JUDGING RESEARCH

The members of the National Commission articulated a set of principles in a brief but remarkably clear document entitled *The Belmont Report*.[7] Subtitled "Ethical Principles and Guidelines for the Protection of Human Subjects of Research," *The Belmont Report* drew on prominent writings in Western philosophy in identifying three basic ethical principles: "Respect for Persons," "Beneficence," and "Justice". This last principle dictates that the benefits and burdens of biomedical research must be distributed equitably in the population — among all racial and ethnic groups, social classes, and females as well as males. The first two principles were explicated as follows.

> Respect for persons incorporates at least two ethical convictions: first, that individuals should be treated as autonomous agents, and second, that persons with diminished autonomy are entitled to protection. The principle of respect for persons thus divides into two separate moral requirements: the requirement to acknowledge autonomy and the requirement to protect those with diminished autonomy.[8]

The leading application of this principle is in the doctrine of informed consent. Failure to obtain voluntary, informed consent from subjects or their legally authorized representatives violates the "respect for persons" principle in the research setting as well as in the context of performing therapy on patients.

The Belmont Report treated beneficence as an obligation, which embraces two general rules: (1) do not harm and (2) maximize possible benefits and minimize possible harms. It is a version of the utilitarian ethical principle, which holds that right actions and practices are those that tend to result in the greatest welfare for the greatest number of people. This type of principle is known as "consequentialist", since it makes the rightness or wrongness of actions a function of their consequences. In contrast, the "respect for persons" principle is nonconsequentialist. The rightness or wrongness of actions judged by this principle depends not on the consequences of the actions but rather, whether they demonstrate respect for the dignity and autonomy of persons.

Applying a nonconsequentialist moral principle would appear to yield a rather different assessment of at least some research involving human subjects. For example, the notion that persons should not be treated as mere things, as instruments to serve the ends or purposes of others, was referred to earlier as a fundamental precept of moral life. This notion is rooted in a moral imperative put forth by the 18th century German philosopher, Immanuel Kant. This imperative states that human beings are never to be treated merely as means but always as ends in themselves. If taken in its strictest sense, this principle might rule out all non-therapeutic research. It would surely prohibit experiments involving individuals who will receive no direct benefit and who lack the capacity to grant informed consent to participate.

However, it has been argued that children who participate in research that does not promise any direct benefits to them might still benefit indirectly. If they are old enough to comprehend the nature of research and the idea that it can help other children in the future, the research subjects themselves may derive the benefit of acting from altruistic motives. Adult subjects of research have been known to acknowledge the motive of wishing to help others as a reason for volunteering to be a subject, and so it is plausible to assume that children whose personality is still in the process of developing can acquire similar motives.

The involvement of children in research in which they do not stand to receive any direct benefit was debated by the National Commission. Some people argued then, and others have continued to argue, that it is unethical to conduct non-therapeutic research on individuals who cannot consent on their own behalf. The ethical principle that can justify the inclusion of nonconsenting subjects in research is the principle of beneficence, which requires acting so as to produce benefits for others. The social utilitarian view of beneficence allows for the possibility of harm to a few so long as those harms are outweighed by substantial benefits to the many.

The National Commission chose this principle as the appropriate standard for judging the acceptability of risks in human experimentation. This necessitates making *risk–benefit assessments* in order to ensure that the anticipated benefits of the research outweigh the risks to subjects. Although the risks are always borne by the subjects, the principle of beneficence allows the benefits to apply to others (including future patients) as well as to the subjects themselves. Researchers thus have an obligation to obtain the most favorable benefit–risk ratio in designing and carrying out research. The National Commission paid particular attention to the application of this ethical principle to research involving children, since children are vulnerable and stand in even greater need of protection than adult subjects of research. As the Commission observed, "Effective ways of treating childhood diseases and fostering healthy developments are benefits that serve to justify research involving children — even when individual research subjects are not direct beneficiaries."[9]

MAKING RISK–BENEFIT ASSESSMENTS

Federal regulations include the following two requirements for IRB approval of research: (1) that risks to subjects are minimized, and (2) that risks to subjects are reasonable in relation to anticipated benefits. This means that an IRB must carry out a risk–benefit analysis for each protocol it reviews. However, making risk–benefit assessments is often not an easy task, whether carried out in the context of providing medical services or in research involving clinical trials. The task is made even harder by the fact that reasonable people disagree both in their evaluations of the magnitude of risks and benefits, and also how to weigh potential risks against expected benefits.

Identifying and assessing risks and benefits has an objective, scientific component and a subjective element that varies with the one who is making the assessment. "Objective" means that agreement can be attained among scientists and researchers based on observations, previous studies, and clinical experience. For example, the identification of the risks and side effects of drugs, the probability of their occurrence, and their severity is based on experience from earlier studies. Once a sufficiently large patient population has been studied, medical scientists should be able to agree on what risks might be expected, how likely they are to occur, and how severe they are in terms of morbidity and mortality. The same is true of benefits, when benefits are taken in a relatively narrow medical sense. The narrow medical sense is best captured by the concept of efficacy: a drug does what it is designed to do — provide a cure, alleviate symptoms, produce a temporary remission, and so on.

There is, moreover, an irreducibly subjective element in risk–benefit assessments. "Subjective" means the insertion of an individual's values, taken in the broadest sense, into the process of assessing risks and benefits and weighing risks against benefits. To take a common example, members of committees that review human subjects research often disagree on the level of risk posed by a particular procedure. The IRB on which I serve has had fierce disagreements over what level of risk to assign to placement of an indwelling urethral catheter in hospitalized 6-year-old boys, or to performing a lumbar puncture on infants.

One study surveyed chairpersons of pediatric departments and directors of pediatric clinical research units in order to find out how pediatricians ranked the level of risk of various procedures commonly used in research. "The results demonstrated serious disagreements among respondents: 14% thought tympanocentesis (puncturing of the ear drum) posed minimal risk or less, 46% classified this as a minor increment over minimal risk, and 40% thought it more than a minor increase."[10] These were not the only disagreements elicited in the survey; "substantial scatter across the categories was the rule rather than the exception throughout the study."[11]

The same mix of objective and subjective elements enters into balancing risks and benefits. That, too, is partly a scientific matter, based on available evidence regarding the probability and magnitude of anticipated risks and benefits; but, it is also a subjective matter. Different people — be they medical scientists, patients, or healthy laypersons — may value the risks and benefits differently. They may consider some risks worth taking in relation to expected benefits while other risks may be viewed as unacceptably high in relation to expected benefits.

Balancing potential risks against expected benefits is always a difficult matter, and is even more so with pediatric patients. That is because adult patients can be permitted to judge for themselves which risks are worth taking, once they have been properly informed by their physician. But in the case of children, it is their parents, in addition to physicians, who are balancing risks against benefits. Although parents can usually be presumed to have their children's best interests at heart, it may be difficult for them to separate their children's interests from their own.

Research involving children requires making the additional distinctions mentioned in the above-noted study of pediatricians' ranking of risks: Does the research carry only "minimal risk"? If it involves more than minimal risk, does the research present the prospect of direct benefit to the children who serve as subjects? If there is no direct benefit and the research involves greater than minimal risk, does the risk represent a "minor increase over minimal risk"?[12] *The Belmont Report* refers to the "difficult ethical problem ... about research that presents more than minimal risk without immediate prospect of direct benefit to the children involved."[13] The rationale that lies behind the "minimal risk" standard is the recognition that children are nonconsenting subjects of research and therefore stand in greater need of protection than consenting adults. In order to derive the overall benefits that may result from pediatric research and at the same time protect pediatric subjects of non-therapeutic research, the "minimal risk" standard was introduced as a safeguard in addition to parental consent and IRB review.

An initial difficulty is how to define "minimal risk". The Federal Regulations contain the following definition: "Minimal risk" means that the risks of harm anticipated in the proposed research are not greater, considering probability and magnitude, than those ordinarily encountered in daily life or during the performance of routine physical or psychological examinations or tests."[14] This definition has been criticized for being too imprecise.[15] In addition, it gives rise to another difficulty: should the risks of daily life be measured against a societal norm of risks children typically face in their everyday activities? Or should those risks be measured against the actual background of minors who are the subjects of the research? It is evident that these two standards may be widely disparate, especially in the case of sensitive research. For example, if the research subjects are adolescents who are using drugs, engaging in behaviors at high risk for acquiring HIV infection, are juvenile offenders, or children who have been physically or sexually abused, the risks they encounter in their daily lives are of considerable magnitude.

Fairness dictates maintaining the same standard of "minimal risk" for all children and adolescents, except where the research being conducted is studying a particular area in which the everyday life or ongoing medical treatment places these children at high risk of harm. The fact that some children live in an inner city area where they are constantly at risk for being hit by stray bullets should not allow them to be placed at higher risk than their suburban counterparts in a study in which children are enrolled. On the other hand, research with minors who have been physically or sexually abused, research with adolescent crack users or intravenous drug users, or sexually active youth at risk for acquiring HIV infection could be based on a higher level of risk of daily life than, say, biomedical research unrelated to the child's risky behavior or situation. In other words, "minimal risk" for minors conforms to a uniform, objective standard of calibrating risks of daily life, except where the research focuses on a medical condition or high-risk behavior of the subjects.

This standard could permit research with minors that involves more than minimal risk yet provides no direct benefit to them, allowing for more than one standard of "minimal risk". However, to use different standards for research depending on the specific characteristics of a subject population is open to the critical charge of manipulating ethical standards to serve the needs of research. How can this be justified without violating the principle of justice, a principle that requires a fair distribution of the benefits and burdens of research?

The answer lies in seeing who will be the expected beneficiaries of this type of research. Since this group of minors is in a class of youth who are subject to high risks, anticipated benefits of the research will accrue to this same group. In explicating the principle of justice in research, *The Belmont Report* states: "Justice demands that .... research should not unduly involve persons from groups unlikely to be among the beneficiaries of subsequent applications...".[16] Conversely, if the only way to provide benefit to members of these groups is to conduct research involving those groups, a higher level of risk may be justified by the prospect of future benefits. Thus the use of different standards of "minimal risk", geared to specific subject populations, does not violate the principle of justice in research, but rather, comports with that principle. It seeks to distribute the risks fairly in virtue of who is likely to benefit from the results of the research.

INFORMED CONSENT AND MINORS' "ASSENT"

Because children are vulnerable, and especially because research might not provide direct benefit to them, the issue of consent to their participation becomes paramount. When adults are subjects of research, they are presumed capable of providing consent on their own behalf. The Respect for Persons principle, which holds that "individuals should be treated as autonomous agents",[17] is geared to the requirement of informed consent. A fuller picture of the basis of this ethical requirement is spelled out in *The Belmont Report*:

> An autonomous person is an individual capable of deliberation about personal goals and of acting under the direction of such deliberation. To respect autonomy is to give weight to autonomous persons' considered opinions and choices while refraining from obstructing their actions unless they are clearly detrimental to others.[18]

At what age does a child become autonomous, in the sense just described? Is an adolescent an autonomous person? The National Commission was silent on this matter. The Respect for Persons principle is intended to apply only to adults. Yet the principle incorporates a second important ethical conviction: "Persons with diminished autonomy are entitled to protection."19 This second ethical conviction is described more fully as follows:

> ... not every human being is capable of self-determination. The capacity for self-determination matures during an individual's life and some individuals lose this capacity wholly or in part because of illness, mental disability, or circumstances that severely restrict liberty. Respect for the immature and the incapacitated may require protecting them as they mature or while they are incapacitated.[20]

Autonomy is the result of cognitive and emotional processes that mature as individuals approach adulthood. Consequently, knowledge about child development might be useful in developing ethical standards for research involving minors. Paternalistic behavior toward infants and young children is ethically justified; indeed, it is ethically obligatory. But since the capacity for self-determination matures during an individual's life, there comes a point at which paternalism exercised by parents, teachers, and other authorities must give way to respect for the minor's autonomy.

It is obvious that infants and very young children lack the capacity to understand the information pertinent to granting informed consent: that they are being asked to participate in research, what the purpose of the research is, the procedures to be done, the risks posed to them by the research, the benefits to themselves or to others, and the alternatives to participation. However, teenagers can be expected to understand at a level equivalent to adult subjects,[21] and children between ages 7 and 12 have the capacity to understand some, but not all of what is involved in being a research subject. The concept of "minors' assent" to participate in research was introduced to denote a simplified version of informed consent.

Prior to 1983, parental informed consent was sufficient for enrollment of a child in research. Federal regulations introduced in that year incorporated the recommendations made by the National Commission in its 1977 report, including the requirement of the "assent" of children over the age of seven, along with parental permission. On this schema, both the permission of the parent and the assent of the child are preconditions to the child's enrollment in the research. This means that parents may not "volunteer" a child without the child's agreement, except in the case of a potentially lifesaving experimental treatment when no other therapy is available. This arrangement "promotes shared decision-making and, in essence, provides independent veto power by parent and minor in matters concerning the minor's research participation."[22] It also shows respect for a child as a developing person, one who may have cogent reasons for not wanting to participate in research. One commentator has proposed that "Dissent from participation or withdrawal from research is always to be honored unless the protocol affords access to a therapeutic intervention that is not otherwise available."[23]

Considerable uncertainty continues to surround the concept of minors' assent: how, precisely, does it differ from consent? Assent is defined in the federal regulations as "a child's affirmative agreement to participate in research."[24] Moreover, "mere failure to object should not, absent affirmative agreement, be construed as assent." How much understanding of a particular research maneuver is required for a child to properly give assent? And how high or low should the child's general cognitive capacity be set for assent to be meaningful? In addition, from an ethical point of view there may be as much cause for concern about children's ability to assent voluntarily as about their understanding of the purposes, risks, and benefits of the research. One author has urged that "in seeking assent, undue advantage should not be taken of the child's developmental limitations related to his or her voluntariness (acquiescence to authority figures and the lack of expression of fulfillment of his or her rights)."[25]

A special circumstance has arisen in the case of parents who do not want their child to know the diagnosis of a serious or fatal illness. This problem has come before my Institutional Review Board several times for children with AIDS, whose parents want them to be enrolled in research but do not want them to learn that they have AIDS. In such circumstances, the information disclosed to the child on the "assent" form may omit the child's diagnosis and substitute, instead, a phrase such as "I have been told that I have an infection caused by a virus that can make me sick."

Although it may be ethically preferable for the child to be informed of a diagnosis of a fatal illness, it is not part of the obligation of a researcher to make the disclosure. Since the researcher's primary activity is not that of clinical care, the obligations are not the same as that of the pediatrician whose sole concern must be for the well-being of the patient. However, when the researcher and the primary-care clinician are one and the same person, obligations to the patient are broadened. The ethical dilemma then becomes one of respecting parental wishes versus obligations to the pediatric patient to disclose information that the pediatrician believes is warranted and in the child's best interest.

EXAMPLES OF ETHICALLY UNSOUND RESEARCH

A much-discussed example of ethically problematic research is the Willowbrook hepatitis study, carried out in the 1960's at the Willowbrook State School, a New York State facility most of whose residents were mentally retarded. The study involved deliberately infecting with hepatitis virus children whose parents consented to their participation. Children who were wards of the state were not included in the studies. The researchers defended the experiment by pointing out that virtually all children enrolled in Willowbrook contracted hepatitis anyway, and that serving as research subjects afforded these children better living conditions — better hygiene, more attention from staff, less crowding — than others in the institution. The researchers wrote:

> It was inevitable that susceptible children would become infected in the institution. Hepatitis was especially mild in the 3- to 10-year age group at Willowbrook. These studies would be carried out in a special unit with optimum isolation facilities to protect the children from other infectious diseases such as shegellosis, and parasitic and respiratory infections which are prevalent in the institution. It should be emphasized that the artificial induction of hepatitis implies a "therapeutic" effect because of the immunity which is conferred.[26]

Despite the defense of the researchers that they were "benefitting" these children by deliberately giving them hepatitis, many people — including physicians — objected that the research design was morally objectionable, and that both the researchers who conducted the study and the parents who consented on behalf of their children made a morally wrong decision. Critics pointed out that unlike other residents of Willowbrook, the children who were subjects in the hepatitis research did not receive protective doses of gamma-globulin that presumably might have lowered the likelihood of acquiring the infection.[27]

There was a long waiting list for Willowbrook, and parents who agreed to enroll their children in the hepatitis study were assured of early admittance. After 1964, no new patients were admitted to Willowbrook because of severe overcrowding; however, the hepatitis research unit continued to enroll children whose parents "volunteered" them for the studies.[28] This raises the question of whether the parents were offered an "undue inducement" to volunteer their children as research subjects. It also serves as a reminder of a point made earlier, namely, the difficulty parents may have in separating their own interests from those of their children.

The consent process was further criticized for the fact that some parents had only been contacted by letter. An even more serious charge was that the consent forms used for the injection read as though the children were to receive a vaccine against the virus.[29]

It may well be true that when judged solely from a consequentialist perspective, the impressive results of the project and its follow-up studies could justify having carried it out. It is probably true that the Willowbrook hepatitis research resulted in significant and positive benefits, both in the knowledge gained and in its eventual application (development of a vaccine for hepatitis). Yet this episode demonstrates the shortcomings of a purely utilitarian perspective in ethics. Values besides that of promoting general welfare must be brought into the moral arena. The judgment that the Willowbrook hepatitis study was an example of unethical research can be defended by appealing to the rights and interests of the children who served as unconsenting experimental subjects.

Another ethical consideration raised by the Willowbrook hepatitis study is the fact that the subjects were institutionalized children. One religious ethicist, who repeatedly questioned the enrollment of children in research that did not directly benefit them, was a staunch critic of the Willowbrook study because the children were in an institution.

> Even if one granted the right of parents to consent for their children to be used in medical investigations having unknown present and future risks to them and promising future possible benefits only for others, it would still be possible to argue that children in institutions and not directly and continuously under the care of parents or relatives should never be so used. If we are not persuaded that because they are *children* children cannot consent (nor should anyone else consent in their behalf) to experiments primarily for the accumulation of knowledge, we at least should be convinced that such experiments ought not to be performed upon children in orphanages, reformatories, or homes for the retarded because they are a captive population.[30]

Although this position appears persuasive, it places too much weight on the fact of institutionalization and insufficient weight on the question of who should give permission for enrollment in research of children who are not living at home with their parents or legal guardians. To disqualify all institutionalized children or all children without parents able to consent on their behalf might be to deny such children the benefits of biomedical research.

This situation has emerged with the advent of AIDS and the fact that research protocols have offered the only or most likely prospect of benefit to children with HIV infection.

CHILDREN WITHOUT PARENTS ABLE TO CONSENT

Special problems arise in the conduct of research involving children who are not in the custody of their biological parents. Although this category of children would normally not receive undue attention as potential research subjects, the advent of AIDS and the quest for therapies to combat the disease has prompted the need for research in pediatric AIDS.

The percentage of HIV-infected children who are not in the custody of their biological parent or parents is known to be high, although precise figures are not available. Estimates from one center with a high prevalence of pediatric AIDS provides a figure of 65–70% of children with HIV infection living with someone other than their biological parents. In the earliest years of the AIDS epidemic, the pediatric AIDS population consisted mostly of infants and children who had received blood transfusions or blood products, such as hemophiliacs. As the demographics of the epidemic have shifted, the majority of infected children are now born of mothers who were intravenous drug users (IVDUs) or who have been sexual partners of IVDUs.

Obtaining consent for investigational drug treatment of HIV-infected children thus poses a myriad of problems, both in theory and in practice. At least four distinct situations exist:

(1) Biological parents are living, but children have been removed from their custody.

(2) Biological parents are no longer living or cannot be located, and children are living with relatives who have not been appointed legal guardians. (Cases in which relatives have become legal guardians are, for purposes of consent to research, identical to those in which children are in the custody of their biological parents.)

(3) Biological parents are not living or cannot be found, and the children have been placed in foster care.

(4) Biological parents are not living or cannot be found, and children are neither in foster care nor with relatives. Some are "boarder babies" living in hospitals, and some may be in congregate care facilities.

Who may grant consent for research with the children in all of these situations, and who should have responsibility to do so?

CHILDREN WITH NONCUSTODIAL LIVING PARENTS

In theory, when biological parents are living, they retain the authority to grant informed consent to research with their children. If they have temporarily lost custody of their children, a child welfare agency assumes responsibility for authorizing medical treatment and research involving such children. But, biological parents are not entirely cut off from the consenting process. The situation is, at the least, confusing, and at worst, can fail to result in the child's best interest being served.

Some ethical and empirical questions about this situation are:

- Even when biological parents retain the legal right to consent for children not in their custody, are they normally requested or required to do so by the supervisory agency?
- If biological parents and the supervisory agency disagree regarding consent to research, whose view should prevail?
- Should the entitlement of parents to decide about research with their children be removed entirely if they have lost custody, even if the loss of custody is viewed as temporary?
- Can bureaucratic entities, such as child protective services or foster care agencies, ever truly be regarded as *in loco parentis* for the purpose of consenting to research? This last question is pertinent to the wide range of situations in which children are not living with their biological parents.
- When children are in foster care but their biological parents are still alive, should the foster parents play any role in the consent process? In some cases, foster parents have become the "psychological" parents of the child. In some cases, foster parents are seeking to adopt the child. In other instances, foster care placement is temporary and the biological parent(s) will regain custody of the child. Do these variations matter with regard to who should have responsibility to consent to research?

CHILDREN LIVING WITH RELATIVES

The situation in which children are living with relatives, often a grandparent, seems easy from an ethical standpoint. The fact that the grandmother or the mother's sister has not been officially appointed as guardian of the child is perhaps a legal barrier, but should not constitute an ethical obstacle to permit the relative to consent to research. The relative has assumed all other responsibilities for the child, and can be presumed to have the child's best interest at heart in precisely the same sense that parents are presumed to act in the child's best interest. What seems truly bizarre is the requirement that the child protective agency be the official consenting party when children are living with caring relatives. Can a bureaucracy ever assume the role of "guardian" of a child in the way that a person who knows the child is able to do?

CHILDREN IN FOSTER CARE

Foster care poses similar problems, but with even more complications. That is because still another layer of bureaucracy is frequently involved: a foster care agency. When children are in foster care, it may be the case that both the foster agency and the governmental bureaucracy must be approached for consent to research. Foster parents are not legally authorized to grant informed consent on behalf of children either for treatment or research. In New York City, for example, the Child Welfare Administration, which oversees all individual foster care agencies, has historically resisted allowing children in foster care to be enrolled in any biomedical research. The bureaucracy had issued a blanket refusal to consent (although that has now changed), and so children were not enrolled in research. That general resistance could be defended by a sound ethical rationale. If a proposed treatment has not been proven to be beneficial, there is good reason to question or disallow the recruitment of children without parents, who would presumably decide in their children's best interest.

But, where there is no "standard" treatment for a disease, as in the case of AIDS, an experimental drug holds out the only hope. Not only does bureaucratic resistance deny that potential benefit to children without parents authorized to consent in their behalf. It also violates the principle of justice in research: The benefits and burdens of biomedical research should be equitably distributed among all classes or groups in society. "An injustice occurs when some benefit to which a person is entitled is denied without good reason or when some burden is imposed unduly."[31]

"BOARDER BABIES" AND CHILDREN IN CONGREGATE FACILITIES

Like the children in the other categories, "boarder babies" and children who have been placed in congregate care facilities have a child protective agency as their legally authorized guardian. But these children lack an adult caregiver who acts as a "psychological" parent or could be a potential adoptive parent. Is it reasonable to think that their bureaucratic guardian could possibly make decisions in their behalf in the way that an individual who knows them can?

The situation that developed as a growing number of children with AIDS became wards of the city or state resulted in a clear need for a mechanism to provide consent for this group of children to enroll in studies. In New York City, after agitation from some pediatricians in the Bronx and other locations with a high prevalence of AIDS, the Child Welfare Administration changed its position. This reversal required instituting some procedures to ensure compliance with the section in the federal regulations dealing with wards of the state or city. Such children could only be involved in research studies if the research is: (1) Related to their status as wards; or, (2) Conducted in schools, camps, hospitals, institutions, or similar settings in which the majority of children involved as subjects are not wards. And, ... the IRB shall require appointment of an advocate for each child who is a ward, in addition to any other individual acting on behalf of the child as guardian or *in loco parentis*.[32] The advocate must be someone who has the background and experience to act in, and who agrees to act in the child's best interests.

At our institution it was decided that we would appoint our own Ward Advocate for pediatric patients. The individual who was asked and agreed to serve as Ward Advocate is a highly regarded pediatrician, well liked by colleagues and trainees, and viewed as both an excellent clinician and a strong advocate of pediatric patients. If implemented properly and conscientiously, this mechanism holds promise for acting in the best interest of children with AIDS who are not in the custody of their parents.

THE ETHICAL CONDUCT OF PEDIATRIC RESEARCH

An example of ethically unacceptable research was proposed a number of years ago in my own institution. One of the very few proposed research projects that was rejected by the

IRB on which I serve because of an unfavorable risk–benefit ratio was a study that required injecting hormones and other drugs into children. The subjects were pre-adolescent and adolescent boys who had been diagnosed as having depression and conduct disorders. At intervals over a period of weeks, the subjects were to be admitted to the hospital and have different drugs injected into them, after which their blood would be examined to see the effect of these drugs on hormones that occur naturally in the body. Each session was to last about four hours, with the boys required to undergo an "overnight fast," with no breakfast in the morning, and to remain lying down until the session ended at 1 p.m. The stated purpose of the research was to learn more about the activity of hormones and neurotransmitters, and the relationship between these and the children's mood and behavior. The study promised no benefit to the children enrolled, but potential contributions to knowledge, which might benefit other children with depression and conduct disorders.

An *ad hoc* committee was formed, chaired by a pediatrician and including another pediatrician, a cancer specialist, a social scientist, and myself. The committee discussed the matter at length, but had no trouble coming to a conclusion. We recommended that the research protocol be rejected on grounds of the poor risk–benefit ratio. Expressing the unanimous view of the group, the chairperson wrote:

> Children are most vulnerable to experimental research. Often their parents are desperate to find out some answer or achieve some fast result and all too unwittingly but willingly submit a child to a research protocol. At the same time, the entire area of obtaining truly informed consent from children leaves many questioning, doubtful aspects. It becomes imperative, therefore, that at least the minimal federal regulations be met when conducting research involving children.

As one noted authority has observed: "To be a child is to be at risk, dependent, and without capacity or authority to decide what is "best" for oneself."[28] To be a child and a subject of biomedical research is to be doubly at risk. Therefore, adults who are properly situated have obligations to seek to ensure that children are not harmed as a result of serving as participants in research, and also that children who might be benefitted have the opportunity to serve as research subjects.

Which adults are properly situated to carry out these obligations? First and foremost, the child's parents, who are uniquely placed to make decisions in the child's interest and who have the authority to grant or refuse permission for the child to serve as a research subject. Also well situated are biomedical researchers and their colleagues who design and carry out research protocols. They have the obligation to minimize risks to subjects, both in the research design and its implementation. Researchers also have the obligation of providing full information to the child's parents, and appropriate information to the child, in clear and understandable language.

Pediatricians who are not themselves researchers have an obligation, when they refer their patients to specialists, to ensure that those pediatric specialists who conduct research are knowledgeable and reputable members of the medical research community. When feasible, the primary pediatrician should also be available to convey to the parents or child information about what the research will involve.

Members of IRBs have a special obligation to pediatric subjects of research. All research protocols involving children should be given full committee review, even if the research maneuvers pose minimal risks, such as blood drawings or routine physical examinations. When the subjects of research are adolescents, IRBs should be sensitive to their concerns about privacy and their need for confidentiality. Especially for research in sensitive areas such as use of drugs or alcohol and sexual behavior, the privacy and confidentiality of adolescent participants must be respected.

If adults in these various situations fulfill their obligations regarding the involvement of children as research subjects, the risks to children are likely to be minimized. Moreover, since research that provides direct benefit to subjects may give sick children a better outcome than that offered by the standard therapy, it is important to remain alert to the opportunity for children to benefit from being participants in research. These efforts require constant vigilance on the part of all adults who have responsibility for protecting the health and well being of our most vulnerable citizens.

References

1. Portions of this chapter are adapted from Macklin, R. (1988). *Mortal Choices: Ethical Dilemmas in Modern Medicine*. Boston: Houghton; Mifflin; and Macklin, R. (1992). Autonomy, beneficence, and child development. In: *Social Research on Children and Adolescents: Ethical Issues*, edited by B. Stanley and J. E. Sieber. Newbury Park, CA: SAGE Publications, pp. 88–105.
2. Kor, E. M. (1992). Nazi experiments as viewed by a survivor of Mengele's experiments. In: *When Medicine Went Mad: Bioethics and the Holocaust*, edited by A. L. Caplan; Totowa, NJ: Humana Press, pp. 3–8. Vigorito, S. S. (1992). A profile of Nazi medicine. In Caplan, op cit. pp. 9–13; Segal, N. L. (1992). Twin research at Auschwitz-Birkenau. In Caplan, op cit. pp. 281–299.
3. National Research Act, Public Law 93–348, July 12, 1974.
4. National Commission for the Protection of Human Subjects of Biomedical and Behavioral Research (1977). *Report and Recommendations: Research Involving Children*. Washington, D.C.: Government Printing Office.
5. Code of Federal Regulations, Title 45, Part 46 — Protection of Human Subjects, revised as of March 8, 1983.
6. 45 CFR 46 Federal Register (January 26, 1981).
7. National Commission for the Protection of Human Subjects of Biomedical and Behavioral Research (1979). *The Belmont Report: Ethical Principles and Guidelines for the Protection of Human Subjects of Research*. Washington, D.C.: Department of Health, Education, and Welfare.
8. Ibid., p. 4.
9. Ibid., p. 4.
10. Freedman, Fuks, and Weijer, p. 15, citing an article by Janosky, J. and Starfield, B. (1981). Assessment of risk in research on children. *J. Pediatr.*, **98**:842–46.
11. Ibid.
12. 45 CFR 46.406.
13. *The Belmont Report*, pp. 4–5.
14. 45 CFR 46.102 (g).
15. Freedman, B., Fuks, A., and Weijer, C. (1993). In loco parentis: minimal risk as an ethical threshold for research upon children. *Hastings Center Report*, **23**:13–19.
16. *The Belmont Report*, p. 5.
17. *The Belmont Report*, p. 4.
18. Ibid.
19. Ibid.

20. Ibid.
21. Weithorn, L. (1983). Children's capacities to decide about participation in research. *IRB: A Review of Human Subjects Research,* **5**:1–5.
22. Grisso, T. (1992). Minors' Assent to Behavioral Research Without Parental Consent. In: *Social Research on Children and Adolescents: Ethical Issues*, edited by B. Stanley and J. Sieber, p. 109.
23. Leiken, S. (1993). Minors' assent, consent, or dissent to medical research. *IRB: A Review of Human Subjects Research*, **15**, p. 6.
24. 45 CFR 46.402.
25. Keiken, p. 6.
26. Krugman, S. and Giles, J. P. (1970). Viral hepatitis: new light on an old disease. *Journal of the American Medical Association*, **212**:1019–1021. Reprinted in: *Moral Problems in Medicine*, (1983) 2nd edition, edited by S. Gorovitz, R. Macklin, A. L. Jameton, J. M. O'Connor, and S. Sherwin. Englewood Cliffs, NJ: Prentice-Hall, p. 603.
27. Faden, R. R. and Beauchamp, T. L. (1986). *A History and Theory of Informed Consent*, p. 164. New York: Oxford University Press.
28. Ibid.
29. Ibid.
30. Ramsey, P. (1970). Children in institutions. *The Patient as Person*. New Haven: Yale University Press. Reprinted in Gorovitz *et al.*, p. 607.
31. *The Belmont Report*, p. 5.
32. 45 CFR 46.409.
33. Goldstein, J. (1982). Medical Care for the Child at Risk. In: *Who Speaks for the Child*? edited by W. Gaylin and R. Macklin. New York and London: Plenum Press, p. 53.

14 Pediatric Practice, Social Responsibility and Physician Advocacy

Irwin Redlener and Susan Grobman

The Children's Health Fund, 317 East 64th Street, New York, New York 10021, USA

INTRODUCTION

In recent years, new insights have raised questions about the boundaries of medical practice and have challenged physicians to re-examine their traditional roles and obligations. While there have always been ethical guidelines and standards regarding conduct in the medical profession, there now seems to be a heightened sensitivity to the relationship between social justice and medicine, in part resulting in an increased interest in serving the common good. The social context of medical practice as well as the responsibilities doctors have to their environment and to the general public are clearly within the domain of the contemporary health professional. According to Sidel, societal needs suggest that if a "medical worker is to be a promoter of health rather than simply a reactor against established disease or disability, part of his work must go beyond traditional medical care."[1]

This chapter will focus on the impact of these considerations and perspectives on the practice of pediatrics. We begin by examining the traditional roles and responsibilities of the physician. We then explore the unique obligations of the pediatrician and the subsequent implications for the practice of pediatrics. It is argued that physicians caring for children have a special obligation to work beyond, as well as within, the traditional "medical model." Furthermore, the question of whether social responsibility should be part of those obligations is analyzed. We conclude with an argument for the incorporation of social responsibility into pediatrics, along with some concrete suggestions for the practicing pediatrician.

Although the profession of pediatrics and the role of pediatricians is emphasized, throughout this chapter the principles, conclusions and recommendations apply equally well to any professional group concerned with the health and well-being of children.

BASIC PRINCIPLES: ETHICS AND PROFESSIONAL RESPONSIBILITY

In the most traditional biomedical model of health care, the primary responsibility of the physician has been to diagnose and treat organic disease in order to restore health or biophysiologic balance. Essential skills to meet such responsibilities are attained through extensive training and practice in well-defined behaviors necessary for a circumscribed range of service and care to patients.[2] However, throughout the course of the professional relationship between physician and patient, especially over the long-term in a primary care setting, unique interactions develop between the provider and the consumer of health care. For instance, patients come to "trust" their physician to provide counsel, propose behavioral changes, organize services that will improve their well-being, eliminate suffering, reduce risk, and so forth.

The physician's medical knowledge and technical skill influence the public's perception of the profession in many ways. Since few laypersons possess much detailed information about their own physiological and anatomical conditions, the perceived ability of the doctor is highly valued. Even when health care was limited to potions and superstitions, doctors were recognized as having a special place in society and a particular authority which was rarely questioned.

The perceptions of the doctor's knowledge affect the doctor–patient relationship. The doctor and the patient have certain expectations (tacit and otherwise) of each other. When people seek treatment from a physician, they render themselves vulnerable because they are ill and because they are actively deferring to the knowledge base or medical expertise of the physician. In submitting to the role of patient, people accept that they should divulge intimate information and, in order to receive the best treatment, *trust* their doctor. As Napodano writes:

> The patient in seeking help does not have a 'gold standard' by which to measure the quality or quantity of the service he is to receive. He must place his trust and confidence in the physician's knowledge and skills and, also, in the physician's interest, commitment, and sincere desire to do what is best for him.[3]

Indeed, when patients visit the doctor there is already an implicit trust grounded in their perception of the medical profession. Over the long-term course of doctor–patient interactions, physicians must sustain this trust by performing with proficiency and compassion, as perceived by the patient.

It can be argued that the knowledge possessed by physicians and the privileged social status and public trust conferred upon them by patients and society, charges them with a professional obligation or duty, to ensure the best care possible for their patients.

Robert Goodin suggests that the vulnerability of patients and families within the doctor–patient relationship creates a special basis for moral responsibility. While it is assumed that the responsibilities we take toward family, friends, clients and patients are dictated by voluntary "self-assumed" choices, contracts, or instincts, what underlies the physician's "*special* responsibilities ... is the peculiar vulnerability of someone else to our actions and choices."[4] [author's emphasis] In the patient–doctor relationship, it is precisely the patient's dependence upon the professional that gives rise to strong obligations on the professional's part.

This responsibility is even greater when lack of political and economic equity in society produces particularly vulnerable populations.[5] Adequate "caring" for such extraordinarily vulnerable patients and families may require the physician to go beyond the traditional (and purist) notion of medical duty. It may necessitate accepting responsibility for social activism, community advocacy and interdisciplinary collaboration. Indeed, the service and care given to patients by their physicians should reflect an understanding of these obligations. How this concept relates to the ethical responsibilities and actual functions of a health care provider will be described later in this chapter.

Recognizing this professional responsibility for the welfare of others, and aware of their special place in society, medical practitioners have typically incorporated into their practice values and attitudes rooted in theories of ethics. Jonsen and Hellegers assert that the ethics of medical care grew out of the general discipline of ethics which emphasized the principles of *autonomy*, *duty*, and a commitment to the *common good*.[6] These provided physicians with a framework within which to relate to their patients.

The belief that physicians should only interact with patients in the most honorable, respectful and egalitarian way arose from the principle of autonomy to which all people should ascribe. Further, the physician's understanding that they must use their unique training to recognize and prevent harm to their patients emerged from the ethical theory of duty. Finally, the commitment to the common good or justice, which has not yet been *formally* incorporated into the medical profession, suggests that there should be institutions to assure the fair and equitable practice of medicine and the provision of care.[7]

As noted, the evolution of ethical standards in medicine was clearly influenced by the essential theories of virtue and duty. However, the "final product", the professional codes of ethics, are distinct and even specific to the special responsibility and powers of the medical profession. Ethical codes and the scope of professional responsibility are continually being redefined by the dynamics among health status and social, economic and environmental conditions. Seen in this way, medical codes are not just guidelines for a physician to follow, but rather tools for moral analysis and self-reflection on his or her role as a doctor. The codes are instrumental in revealing to the physician "not how [people] do in fact behave, but how in principle they should behave" within the scope of their professional work.[8]

Codes and Oaths: The Old and the New

Since Hippocrates, doctors have described, organized and sworn to various sets of vows and behavioral conduct. These codes have been powerful indicators of what physicians have considered to be the prevailing values of the profession. Selections from the Oath of Hippocrates demonstrate a strong regard for the principles of virtue and duty in the doctor–patient interaction:[9]

- I will use treatment to help the sick, according to my ability and judgement, but never with a view to injury and wrong-doing.
- I will keep holy both my life and my art.
- And whatsoever I shall see or hear in the course of my profession, as well as outside my profession, ... I will never divulge, holding such things to be holy secrets.

In 1948, the World Medical Association, in another attempt to articulate the proper responsibilities of the physician, "modernized" the Hippocratic Oath with the Oath of

Geneva.[10] Although the language in the latter oath is clearly updated, the underlying principles continue to reflect the traditional notions about the role of the doctor in the doctor–patient interaction.[11]

A major change in conventional medical ethics is not evident until the revision of the American Medical Association's "Principles of Medical Ethics" in 1957. In contrast to the principles and published codes adopted by their predecessors, the AMA's declaration includes a reference to the community.[12] It states:

> The honored ideals of the medical profession imply that the responsibility of the physician extend not only to the individual, but also to society, and these responsibilities deserve his interest and participation in activities that have the purpose of improving both the health and the *well-being of the individual and the community.*[13] (author's emphasis)

The principles of the AMA represent a progression in ethical thought by the medical profession. The inclusion of the "community" signifies an important departure from the somewhat narrow view that physicians need only be responsible for their individual patients. Additionally, since medicine had consistently favored the good of the individual, this reference suggests the beginnings of a social consciousness about the "common good" in the medical community.[14]

This, indeed, is a realization that the fundamental values of the practice of medicine encompass serious and deliberate attention to the "common good", as well as to the good of individual patients.

THE CURRENT SCOPE OF MEDICAL PRACTICE AND THE SPECIAL PERSPECTIVE OF PEDIATRICS

The evolution of ethical standards in medicine and the formalization of codes which define those standards underscore the notion that physicians have appropriate and legitimate roles that extend beyond the one-to-one, doctor–patient practice dynamic. This may be particularly true for health professionals who work with pediatric populations. In fact, if the historical underpinnings of duty, virtue, and professional obligation are to be met, the pediatric physician must be concerned about all factors which affect children's health, including the external conditions of the family and the community at large.

What are the implications for the practicing physician if it is understood that the physician has an ethical responsibility to improve the health and well-being of the *community* as well as the individual? How do such considerations relate to the practice of medicine and specifically to the practice of pediatrics?

To answer these questions, it might be helpful to examine how pediatricians have responded to this ethical mandate to serve the common good and further how they can incorporate notions of social justice within the scope of practice.

Historically, information conveyed in pediatric textbooks, generally fell under two categories: (1) the description, diagnosis and treatment of diseases of childhood, and (2) an array of general advice on non-disease issues like infant feeding and suggestions for parents interested in "behavioral control" of their children. As late as 1950, even leading textbooks of pediatrics such as *Nelson's Textbook of Pediatrics* offered little overview of the field. Indeed, most early pediatric textbooks described no real social issues, environmental concerns or special advocacy roles for pediatric practitioners. Additionally, no general sense of the meaning of professional responsibility to the individual or the community was presented.

While there have been numerous instances where new knowledge or information brought changes in the scope of medical practice, those changes have mostly influenced the way physicians treat biomedical conditions. For example, the discovery of bacterial pathogens and the subsequent development of antibiotic therapy led to profound changes in medical practice. The realization that contaminated water could lead to cholera epidemics opened the door for clinicians and public health specialists to recommend relevant precautions to patients and urge public policy measures that would safeguard the reservoirs.

But, how do new approaches — whether surgical procedures or public health measures — become accepted within the scope of medical practice? The fact is that the more consistent a "new idea" is with the "traditional biomedical model", the more easily it is incorporated into an expanded version of medical practice.

Many pediatricians, even now, prefer a more limited and traditionally "medical" range of professional work. Although an argument will be made that *all* pediatricians should actively work within the larger context of a child's existence — including the family, the community, and the environment — not all practitioners would agree that such principles apply to the structure and content of their particular practice.

Unfortunately, when the etiology (and solution) of a problem which affects the health and well-being of children is perceived as falling too far outside the classic medical model, physicians have greater difficulty broadening their scope of practice. Thus issues such as securing access to comprehensive care for all children or regulating industries that contaminate the water supply seem to have only a distant and detached relevance to the actual professional work of most physicians.

Yet, perhaps more than other practitioners, pediatricians have an ethical responsibility which spans both medical and social agendas. Since children have less of a voice in changing adverse conditions in their environment, the responsibility of a pediatrician to a child is particularly compelling. A pediatrician who is treating a child injured in an auto accident, needs to be concerned about car safety modalities available to, or required for, families. Managing a patient with lead poisoning is incomplete with standard medical therapy (e.g., chelation) alone. Physicians must be concerned about the origin of the exposure to lead, the conditions of the family's housing and the availability of abatement programs.

A narrow biomedical lens excludes important social issues which have a direct impact on the health and well-being of children and may hamper complete diagnosis or effective intervention.

Sia makes a strong case for incorporating a real social policy focus in children's health systems. Not only are social problems (such as exposure to violence, drugs and teen pregnancy) more prominent in recent years, but public sector programs to deal with these concerns are seemingly less available.[15]

Such social conditions produce compelling pressure for re-examining the child health professional's role in, and responsibility for, *directly* addressing a broad range of relevant

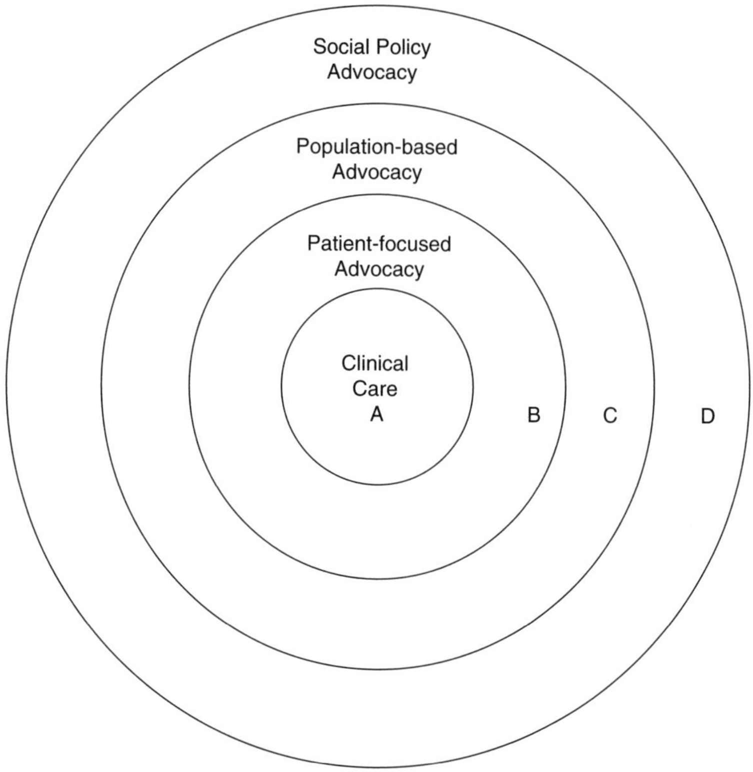

Figure 14.1 Illustrates the possible areas of professional work and advocacy in contemporary pediatrics.

social and environmental conditions. Physical and social scientists may have more specialized technical information than do pediatricians. Politicians may know more about policy development. But, no other group has more expertise than pediatricians in understanding the consequences of adverse conditions upon children. This knowledge per se, as underscored earlier, entails a serious obligation to act in socially responsible ways *within* the scope of professional practice.

The central area of the circle represents the pediatrician's traditional clinical involvement in preventive care, diagnosis, and curative health care. The second ring, labeled "Patient Focused Advocacy", refers to the role of the physician in securing for *specific* patients, need-based entitlement or psychosocial and educational services which are outside of basic medical care. The third circle in the diagram, "Population Based Advocacy", represents the work of the provider in ensuring basic access, and needed services for *large groups of children* who are *not necessarily under his/her direct care and/or responsibility*. Finally, the last ring of the diagram signifies involvement by a pediatrician in the public policy decisions that will have a significant impact on the health and well-being of *all* children.

The Medical Model

The "core" of the concentric circles represents the fundamental or traditional biomedical functions of pediatricians. The behaviors at this level of work are to elicit pathology (in the biomedical sense) and treat the patient with relevant pharmacological or physical interventions. The goal is to restore health or improve bio-physiologic balance.

Sometimes a patient presents to the physician with symptoms which require evaluation or diagnosis. Physical examinations, laboratory testing or observation may contribute relevant information dictating an appropriate course of intervention. In other instances, patients *without* symptoms present to the physician, but routine screening procedures reveal unexpected abnormalities. Such findings may prompt a series of further interventions, all consistent with the classic medical model.

Simply stated, the essence of the education and training of physicians has to do with developing competence in the prevention, detection and treatment of pathology. Physicians need to be good analytic medical diagnosticians, concerned about patients' welfare and skilled in the application of appropriate treatments. These are the essential core of aptitudes of a physician.

Confident and successful fulfillment of the basic medical role enhances esteem and credibility of the health professional as a capable advocate. Pediatricians and other physicians must be able to perform these traditional core functions effectively, no matter how much they also function in the outer rings of advocacy and social policy.

The Outer Rings: Pediatricians as Advocates

Many pediatricians and child health professionals already function well beyond the inner core of basic direct medical care. In most practice settings, it is difficult to ignore the inexorable link between child health and a wide range of familial and social issues. Perhaps without recognizing or defining their work as "advocates", pediatricians naturally gravitate to a larger scope of responsibility, particularly as it pertains to their own patients.

For some professionals, movement out through the concentric rings of expanding advocacy is a gradual process. It may take time, experience and professional maturation to prompt an individual pediatrician to move significantly beyond the traditional (and familiar) concentration within the medical model.

A specific case situation may help to illustrate the relationship between professional roles and the levels of responsibility which could be assumed by pediatricians.

Problem: Head Injury

Biomedical Sphere

A 9-year-old boy presents to the pediatrician following a fall from a bicycle. No helmet was worn. There was no history of loss of consciousness or other neurological symptoms. There is reported "injury" to the right arm with, according to the mother, limitation of movement at the elbow. General and neurological examinations are found to be normal. There is full range of motion of the right arm with no evidence of fracture. The physician reassures the parent and child and sends them home.

Review of the office records indicates that the child has not had a routine health maintenance visit since age 5 and has not had a measles booster shot.

Sociomedical Sphere: Expanded Vision of Relevant Issues

The mother comments that she is "happy nothing else is needed because my husband lost his job and we don't have any health insurance." Further history reveals that this is the child's third fall from a bicycle, none of which previously had resulted in serious injury. All falls have occurred near the child's home at a particular intersection where pot-holed pavement, lack of sidewalk and a downed stop sign are hazardous for bicycle riders.

The physician also learns that the child does not use a bicycle helmet because the parents believe "they are too expensive and don't do much good anyway." Helmets are not mandatory by law in the state.

An analysis of this medical encounter demonstrates the range of potential professional intervention available to the pediatrician. A functional problem list is constructed in Table 14.1.

The most obvious problems are those which might appear in a traditional medical record. Problem #1, "injury", could be handled by an acute care physician in a typical episodic health care environment, such as a hospital emergency service or walk-in center. Most pediatricians, on the other hand, practice in the setting of a comprehensive primary care service where continuity, health maintenance and screening are components of competent medicine.

While the emergency medicine physician might fulfill his/her professional responsibilities by only "handling" problem #1, this by itself would be clearly an insufficient

Table 14.1 Working problem list for case of child with head injury; includes "traditional" bio-medical, psychosocial and public policy concerns. Some would consider all of this under responsibility of pediatrician.

LEVEL	PROBLEM	ACTION DESCRIPTION	INTERVENTION
A.	1. Injury	reassurance	medical, episodic
	2. no helmet use	anticipatory guidance	medical, comprehensive
	3. immunization delay	schedule visit	medical, comprehensive
B.	4. street hazard	complain to city	patient advocacy
	5. no helmet law	work for passage	population advocacy
	6. no health insurance	work for universal health insurance	policy advocacy

intervention for the child health specialist. The standard of care for pediatricians would include attention being paid to problem #2, advising the family on the use of helmet protection and problem #3, making sure that regular visits and the immunization schedules were adhered to by the child.

However, the physician must also look to the larger social and political environment of his patient. This is particularly important for understanding the etiology and successfully managing certain aspects of the case in question. *Why* have there been multiple falls? Possibilities range from poor road conditions (problem #4), to a lack of effective signs, and the like. *Why* is the family not bringing the child in for routine care? The answer relates to the economic barriers faced by the family and the more general problems of access to health services in a country without universal health insurance and health care access (problem #6).

In addition to the necessity for understanding the etiologic substrata of sociomedical problems, it is equally important to move beyond the pure medical model in order to design an appropriate intervention strategy. Clearly, the "treatment" of street hazards and the interventions to ensure universal access to health care are not related to pharmaceutical or surgical procedures. Effective solutions for such problems require analysis and actions which go well beyond the biomedical model. If conducted appropriately, a broader range of traditional and expanded roles may yield profoundly positive consequences for the patient in the above-cited case, as well as for many other children who are personally unknown to the health professional.

But, why should the pediatrician assume a greater range of general health responsibility for the patient under these circumstances? The compelling answer is that the modern definition of pediatrics, as underscored by the standard of care throughout the nation and as articulated by the more prominent pediatric professional organizations, has established this larger practice territory as acceptable and appropriate.

But the question remains: how far does the legitimate role of a pediatrician actually extend?

The answer may be: *as far as necessary to ensure the health and well-being of children.* To fully understand the "real world" implications of this answer it is necessary to explore the various levels of physician advocacy and the concept of "extended expertise".

Patient-focused Advocacy

Many (if not most) pediatricians accept some roles on behalf of their own patients that leads them well outside the confines of the examining room interaction. For instance, helping children with physical or learning disabilities obtain special considerations or placements in school is commonplace. Or, in the example of the child with multiple bicycle falls, a letter or call urging municipal action to correct the hazardous intersection would be entirely "in the line of duty".

Functioning in these ways may be termed "patient-focused advocacy", referring to actions outside the realm of the traditional medical model, but on behalf of *one's own specific patient.* Some might argue that the pediatrician is not an expert in schools or street repair and therefore should not enter these areas of intervention. This is countered, however, by a more dominant professional mandate to act in the best interests of your patients' health and well-being, even if it means acting outside of the biomedical arena.

Another part of the answer raises the questions of precisely who has "expertise", and how the physician could gain access to special bodies of knowledge. Some pediatricians develop expertise in assessing learning disabilities and managing relevant school and educational aspects of these problems. Other physicians become expert in housing policies and the shelter system because they work with families who are homeless. Such areas of "extended expertise" are necessary for the providers to deliver complete and comprehensive care *to their specific patients.*

Even if physicians did not want to invest to the extent of personally developing an area of extended expertise, such a decision would certainly not preclude actively working with those who do possess the needed skills or information. Pediatricians and primary care providers regularly function as "gatekeepers", coordinating and organizing medical subspecialty expertise on behalf of their patients. There is no important difference in working with non-medical experts, particularly when the goal is to prevent injury or illness or enhance the well-being of one's own patients.

Population-focused Advocacy

Sometimes options are available that will reduce risk, improve health or general conditions for a particular class or group of patients, not limited to those in the specific practice of a particular provider. In the case of the bicycle accident with head injury, the existence of a state-wide law mandating the use of helmets for all children might have considerably reduced the risk for the individual patient cited above. But, the focus of concern and benefit should be much broader.

In this circumstance, the pediatrician easily justifies an interest in working on the development and adoption of legislation mandating the use of appropriate head protection *for all children* who ride bicycles on public streets. Such a bill, if successfully passed, would substantially reduce the risk of serious injuries from bicycle accidents for the population as a whole. Working on such legislative initiatives is professionally legitimate.

Such participation is welcomed and seen as appropriate by lawmakers, the press and the public at large. For instance, Robert Sanders, M.D., the Tennessee pediatrician who was instrumental in the passage of the state's mandated car seat legislation, received wide acclaim for his efforts. His legislative activities clearly served as a model for other health professionals.

Social Policy Advocacy

At the outer ring of health professional advocacy, change is sought on the higher levels of public policy. Decisions and actions at this level broadly affect large segments of the population. While such initiatives generally address sweeping changes in public policy, they ultimately affect individual patients in the provider-advocate's practice. Successful advocacy of this nature may involve long-term involvement in the legislative process, in grassroots organizing and with the media. Although the outcome may be highly relevant to broad aims of medical practice, the work involved in this kind of activity will often be characterized as "political".

A current example of important public policy debate concerns the issue of national health reform. Overall health expenditures currently amount to more than 1/7 of the U.S. economy. Even so, more than 39 million Americans are without health insurance coverage; tens of millions of others have inadequate coverage.

One related point which is particularly troubling for the pediatricians is the fact that children now account for as many as 12 million of the uninsured.[16] Child health providers concerned about access to care for children and informed about the necessity of scheduled preventive care and health screening, have compelling reasons to work actively for universal coverage and the elimination of fiscal barriers which interfere with access to care.

In the example of the child with injuries related to the bicycle accident, lack of health insurance and an apparent inability to pay directly for care resulted in a lack of health maintenance visits, lack of age-specific anticipatory guidance and under-immunization. For many pediatricians, such real-life patient situations are sufficient cause to "become politically involved". The support of national efforts to secure universal coverage and systemic health reform, has become an entirely legitimate activity in the view of many physicians, even if this entails seemingly partisan political activities.[10]

If there is a commitment to good access to quality care for all children, one should consider a pediatrician to be obligated to participate in the efforts to attain universal access for all children.

Personally and professionally, raising public awareness, influencing officials and policymakers, and becoming an effective advocate for children's issues are rewarding and fulfilling modalities for the committed pediatrician.

De Facto Advocacy

In reality, many pediatricians are simply not comfortable in the active arena of public policy changes. Some, by reason of practice logistics, financial needs or professional commitments, are unable or unwilling to function in the role of social advocate. Yet these same physicians may still feel a personal, ethical or moral commitment to work toward the goal that all children should receive high quality health care.

In lieu of active advocacy to secure universal access to health care for all children, pediatricians have a second option: *reach out to take medically underserved or unserved children into your own practice arrangement.* This is a limited but effective expression of an essential social principle of modern pediatrics: *all children* should have access to comprehensive children's health services.

In fact, until universal access is firmly in place in the United States, the moral obligation is clear for pediatricians. Seeking ways to provide direct health services to children who are otherwise unable to secure on-going access is what might be termed "*de facto* advocacy" and should be recognized as such.

However, this approach should not be seen as an adequate *substitute* for being active advocates for universal coverage and national health reform. Remember that 12 million children do not have health insurance coverage; several million others are insufficiently covered. Active social policy advocacy remains very much needed because no amount of charitable outreach by individual practitioners could solve this problem in the absence of mandated coverage and access to health care for all children.

GUIDE TO SOCIAL PRACTICE

Societal needs have prompted a re-examination of traditional medical ethics and practice. Today, physicians increasingly recognize that deteriorating social conditions further complicate already serious medical problems. The need to diagnose and appropriately treat a multitude of current medical problems requires that physicians broaden their scope of practice beyond the classic biomedical framework. For instance, the complete care and treatment of a child with lead poisoning must include a thorough investigation of housing conditions and nutritional status. Professional responsibility challenges the physician to accept a more comprehensive role in order to have the greatest impact on the overall health status of a patient. It further dictates that physicians pursue a broader agenda — caring for their individual patients as well as for children and society in general.

Such a role, however, needs to be seen as a "usual and accepted" area of responsibility for *all* pediatricians. Since it is impossible to extricate the biomedical factors from the social–political context of many childhood health problems, pediatricians must be able to see the "big picture" and work with the entire range of relevant etiologic issues and beneficial interventions.

But what are the actual advocacy behaviors appropriate for physicians? Some of these behaviors are everyday actions for pediatricians who regularly intervene on behalf of their patients. Speaking out in the community, communicating with schools and public agencies and even attempting to "educate" elected representatives about particular issues are common professional activities for many physicians.

The following offers more specific ways in which pediatricians and other child health professionals can function as effective advocates for patients and children in general:

1. **Become knowledgeable about non-medical resources for children in the community.** This means knowing what services are available and how referrals to appropriate agencies are organized, managed and followed-up. Current lists should be maintained in the office along with key personal contacts. Referrals can become easier and more comfortable as the physician becomes known to and trusted by relevant individuals and agencies.

2. **Reach out to community-based referral resources.** Pediatricians can do more than simply refer patients for special services. There may be opportunities to interact more directly with the resource program by, for example, participating in on-site case conferences. Schools, developmental centers, head-start programs and a wide range of other special services for children are often able to make excellent use of the expertise and skills of a concerned child health professional. Volunteering to assist such programs can facilitate the communication between the resource service and the referring physician community.

3. **Find opportunities to address community groups.** Individual physicians can become highly effective communicators and offer their time to parent groups, community leaders and service organizations for public speaking opportunities, memberships on committees or service in an advisory role.

4. **Join regional or national "issue initiatives".** Depending on the pediatrician's particular interests, there are many opportunities to join advocacy groups dealing with virtually any important issue from environmental concerns to public health education. A physician can also be an active catalyst in the development of a new issue-focused initiative.

5. **Learn about and communicate with local, state and national elected officials representing your area who are dealing with issues of particular concern.** The impact that individual citizens can have by contacting elected officials can not be overstated. Such one-to-one contact is often even more effective when it is initiated by a physician or child health provider. Letters and calls should be specific and should conclude with a question or particular request that compels an appropriate response from the official.

6. **Attend conferences and programs designed to increase advocacy and communication skills.** Such courses are readily available. Organizations like the Children's Defense Fund and the American Academy of Pediatrics have excellent programs available on a regular basis.

7. **Join relevant organizations.** Active membership in the American Academy of Pediatrics, the Ambulatory Pediatric Association, Physicians for Human Rights, The American Public Health Association, etc., can formally connect the individual physician to a defined organizational agenda. The single voice is greatly amplified by joining the loud and well organized chorus of a larger group.

8. **Utilize the Media.** There are many opportunities here. Newspapers publish letters to the editor and so-called "op-ed" articles. Local and regional papers frequently publish submissions from physicians. Likewise, radio and television talk shows provide physicians with a forum to speak out on a range of issues.

9. **Contact Educational Organizations.** Promote their awareness that the curricula of medical schools and of child health professional training programs should include an emphasis on the evolving role of the physician as advocate.

CONCLUSION

The experience of physician–advocates demonstrates that doctors do have a significant role in working for change on behalf of their patients and the larger community. This capacity to make a real and lasting difference should not be underestimated. There are ample ethical, historical and practical reasons for developing an advocacy agenda within the range and scope of any physician's practice.

Society has come to expect pediatricians and their colleagues to participate in the societal debates and decisions which affect the health and well-being of children. The modern pediatrician must use his or her expertise and insight as a guide for working towards the amelioration of conditions which are unjust or conditions which can lead to increased health risk or decreased access to care for children. It is precisely this expanded scope of work that may define the practice of pediatrics into the next century.

References

1. Sidel, V. W. (1972). Medical Ethics and Socio-Political Change. In: *The Teaching of Medical Ethics*, edited by R. Veatch, W. Gaylin & Councilman Morgan. Hastings-On-Hudson: Institute of Society, Ethics and the Life Sciences, pp. 29–37.
2. Napodano, R. J. (1986). *Values in Medical Practice*. New York: Human Sciences Press, pp. 27–29.
3. Napodano, R. J. (1986). *Values in Medical Practice*. New York: Human Sciences Press, p. 28.
4. Goodin, R. E. (1985). *Protecting the Vulnerable: A Reanalysis of Our Social Responsibilities*. Chicago: University of Chicago Press, pp. 205–206.
5. Goodin, R. E. (1985). *Protecting the Vulnerable: A Reanalysis of Our Social Responsibilities*. Chicago: University of Chicago Press, p. 206.
6. Jonsen, A. R., Hellegers A. E. (1976). Conceptual Foundations for an Ethics of Medical Care. In: *Ethics and Health Policy*, edited by R. Veatch and R. Branson. Massachussets: Ballinger Publishing Company, p. 19.
7. Jonsen, A. R., Hellegers, A. E. (1976). Conceptual Foundations for an Ethics of Medical Care. In: *Ethics and Health Policy*, edited by R. Veatch and R. Branson. Massachussets: Ballinger Publishing Company, p. 22.
8. Jonsen, A. R., Hellegers, A. E. (1976). Conceptual Foundations for an Ethics of Medical Care. In: *Ethics and Health Policy*, edited by R. Veatch and R. Branson, p. 18. Massachussets: Ballinger Publishing Company, p. 18
9. Selections from the Hippocratic Corpus. In Ethics in Medicine: Historical Perspectives & Contemporary Concerns, edited by J. R. Reiser, A. J. Dyck & W. J. Curran. Massachussets: MIT Press, pp. 5–6.
10. Sidel, V. W. (1972). Medical Ethics and Socio-Political Change. In: *The Teaching of Medical Ethics*, edited by R. Veatch, W. Gaylin & Councilman Morgan. Hastings-On-Hudson: Institute of Society, Ethics and the Life Sciences, p. 31.
11. World Medical Association (1948). Declaration of Geneva. In: *Ethics in Medicine: Historical Perspectives & Contemporary Concerns*, edited by J. R. Reiser, A. J. Dyck & W. J. Curran. Massachussets: MIT Press, p. 37–38.
12. Sidel, V. W. (1972) Medical Ethics and Socio-Political Change. In *The Teaching of Medical Ethics*, edited by R. Veatch, W. Gaylin & Councilman Morgan, p. 33. Hastings-On-Hudson: Institute of Society, Ethics and the Life Sciences.
13. Jonsen, A. R., Hellegers, A. E. (1976) Conceptual Foundations for an Ethics of Medical Care. In *Ethics and Health Policy*, edited by R. Veatch and R. Branson, p. 19. Massachussets: Ballinger Publishing Company.
14. Jonsen, A. R., Hellegers, A. E. (1976) Conceptual Foundations for an Ethics of Medical Care. In *Ethics and Health Policy*, edited by R. Veatch and R. Branson, p. 19. Massachussets: Ballinger Publishing Company.
15. Sia, C. C. J. (1992) The Medical Home: Pediatric Practice and Child Advocacy in the 1990's. *Pediatrics*, **90** **(3)**, 419–423.
16. Cartland, J. D. C., Yudkowsky, B. K. (1993) State Estimates of Uninsured Children. *Health Affairs*, **12** **(1)**, 144–151.
17. Employee Benefit Research Institute (1993), *Sources of Health Insurance and Characteristics of the Uninsured*. Brief # 133.

Index